T0249936

Psychoanalysis, Violence and Rage-Type Murder

Many people who commit 'rage-type' murders have no history of violence. Using psychoanalytic theory and a number of case studies, this book isolates key psychological factors that appear to help explain why such acts of extreme violence occur.

Starting from a psychoanalytic standpoint, *Psychoanalysis, Violence and Rage-Type Murder* argues for a pluralistic approach to understanding aggression, and claims that the origins of aggression have no single source or cause. Drawing broadly on psychological, criminological and psychoanalytic research the author outlines the clinical features of the act and explores the possible role that psychopathology and personality might play in the build-up to murder.

These observations raise a number of questions about the so-called 'normality' of the individual alongside the capacity to commit murder, and how we might understand the stability of such offenders. *Pyschoanalysis, Violence and Rage-Type Murder* will be of great interest to psychotherapists, forensic psychotherapists, psychoanalysts, psychologists, criminologists and health care workers.

Duncan Cartwright is a Senior Lecturer at the School of Psychology, University of Durban-Westville, South Africa. Part of his clinical work is dedicated to the assessment and treatment of violent offenders using psychoanalytic principles.

Psychoanalysis, Violence and Rage-Type Murder

Murdering minds

Duncan Cartwright

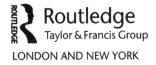
Routledge
Taylor & Francis Group

LONDON AND NEW YORK

First published 2002 by Brunner-Routledge

This edition published 2014 by Routledge
27 Church Road, Hove, East Sussex BN3 2FA
711 Third Avenue, New York, NY 10017, USA

*Routledge is an imprint of the Taylor & Francis Group,
an informa business*

Typeset in Times by Regent Typesetting, London

Paperback cover design by Terry Foley at Anú Design

British Library Cataloguing in Publication Data
A catalogue record for this book is available from the British
Library

Library of Congress Cataloging in Publication Data
Cartwright, Duncan, 1968–
    Psychoanalysis, violence, and rage-type murder : murdering
    minds / Duncan Cartwright.
        p.cm.
    Includes bibliographical references and index.
    ISBN 1-58391-201-0 (hbk) – ISBN 1-58391-202-9 (pbk.)
        1. Psychoanalysis. 2. Violent crimes–Psychological aspects.
3. Murder–Psychological aspects. 4. Criminal psychology. I. Title.

RC506.C315 2002
616.89'17–dc21

2002066748

ISBN 978-1-583-91201-0 (hbk)
ISBN 978-1-58391-202-7 (pbk)

For Gabriel and Nina

Contents

Preface

This book emerges out of my therapeutic work with violent offenders and subsequent doctoral research aimed at exploring the nature and quality of object relations in rage-type murderers. In treating violent offenders, I grew interested in particular intrapsychic factors that appeared linked to violent behaviour. I was also intrigued by how these differed depending on the type of violence displayed. From here my interest grew towards a particular group of offenders who had committed aberrant acts of extreme violence but lacked an often expected history of violence. They also did not display typical psychopathic characteristics and often lived apparently 'normal' lives. In treating rage offenders I had become aware of a number of similarities between cases, especially related to the type of defensive organization adopted and their general approach to conflict.

In order to explore this further, I initiated a research project on a group of such offenders who had been convicted of rage-type murder, the ultimate rage crime. All offenders were male, displaying no history of violence or criminal activity prior to the act. All had been cleared of any neurological impairment and were selected only if they had an IQ that fell within, or above, normal range scores.

The research conducted here was essentially applied psychoanalytical research. Each offender underwent an intensive interviewing process using the Psychoanalytic Research Interview (Cartwright, 2000), an approach developed to explore intrapsychic processes and unconscious meaning derived from core narratives of the interview. The Thematic Apperception Test, the Rorschach and court reports were also used as corroborating sources of evidence in the research process. For the purposes of this book I have selected a number of typical cases to illustrate my broader observations. I have chosen to concentrate on interview and therapeutic accounts and only draw on court records and projective tests where needed to support a particular claim. Some of the details of cases explored have been omitted or changed to protect the confidentiality of the offender and associated others. However, none of the omitted or changed detail alters the essential nature of the cases considered.

In investigating rage offences I have restricted myself to considering only male offenders. Clearly, violence of this kind is not restricted to men, but such attacks are far less frequently committed by women. More importantly, rage attacks committed by women appear to be motivated by different intrapsychic, inter-personal and social factors that require a separate investigation. It is primarily for this reason that I restrict my observations to male offenders.

In considering rage-type violence from an intrapsychic perspective, I in no way wish to diminish the importance of the social, biological or neuropsychological contributions to this field of study. There is no doubt that these factors, depending on the type of violence being considered, have varying roles to play in explaining how violence is precipitated. Although situational elements will be considered here in terms of their impact on the internal world of the individual, the scope of this work does not permit extended consideration of such factors. In this sense it is clear to me that this book provides only partial answers to the problems discussed.

Although this book emerges, in part, from my work as a psychoanalytic therapist, I devote very little space here to treatment concerns and issues of technique. I only make a few comments in the concluding chapter about the implications of my findings for treatment. The present book aims more at under-standing the nature of rage-type violence within the context of the offender's personality. In this way, I see it as preparatory discussion for future considerations related to management, intervention and technique.

Foreword

This is an important book on an important topic. Violent crime has been a focus of concern for social science since its inception, but surprisingly, important psychoanalytic approaches to violence have been far fewer than other perhaps socially less important topics. There may be many reasons for this, including the relative lack of clinical experience of many psychoanalytic clinicians with individuals who are actually capable of violent acts, let alone an act as grave as murder. Rage-type murder has become a focus of public concern, with school shootings in the United States and more recently in Germany. Does a psychoanalytic understanding of the mind have anything to contribute to the questions that these events have raised in the public mind?

The approach taken by Cartwright's scholarly examination of the topic is rooted in an object relations understanding of personality. This is perhaps the first psychoanalytic model since the death of Freud around which there is a degree of consensual acceptance in the psychoanalytic community. Within an object relations framework, the mind is seen as made up of relationship representations, principally self–other relationships, where relationship to aspects of the other may be privileged and separately represented. The lack of integration between images of the other and the experienced relationship to that image is seen as at the root of personality disturbance.

Cartwright uses this model elegantly and in a scholarly way. The puzzle he presents to us is the individual who appeared to live a normal and even good life until provoked into murder by events which may superficially appear almost inconsequential. Cartwright brings the psychoanalytic perspective to bear on these observations and shows how a specific personality type may be particularly vulnerable to such ultimately destructive attacks of rage. He links the personality structure to borderline functioning in a highly original and intriguing way, using the concept of the 'narcissistic exoskeleton' – an apparently stable personality characterized by a particular kind of defensive splitting to keep idealized good objects and an internalized bad object system apart. There are evident links here to Winnicott's concept of the false self, but it is a self that is genuinely experienced as outside of the self-structure.

The model proposed provides a good phenomenological account of many aspects of violent crime, in particular the dissociative experiences linked with rage-type murder and the lack of remorse experienced by murderers who strangely continue to feel that they are not responsible for the act they actually committed. The cause of the murder is the collapse of narcissistic defences, triggered by events or actions which at times have only subtle links to these defensive structures. Cartwright is in agreement with perhaps the most evocative psychoanalytic writer in this field, Gilligan, who has placed the experience of shame at the very centre of his theory of violence. The relief which follows the murder should not be mistaken for a drive discharge; it is an ephemeral internal state created by the fantasy that the murderous action has achieved an evacuation and destruction of shameful 'bad' parts of the self.

There is a great deal more to this book than a persuasive theory of murderous violence. It provides a scholarly review of psychoanalytic contributions to this field, well integrated with epidemiological findings on the one hand and the historical evolution of psychoanalytic ideas on the other. It is also a clinical book, with pragmatic recommendations for those working with such individuals. Using the work of Meloy, Ogden and others Cartwright recommends in treating these patients that the therapy should work towards getting the patient to be able to see a 'third position' and entertain the possibility of alternative interpretations to their own. Cartwright's approach is a combination of object relations and relational technique: it is both theoretically coherent and intuitively appealing. Altogether the book is an extremely valuable contribution to our understanding of what is undoubtedly one of the greatest puzzles that faces any theory of human behaviour. How can we have the propensity to kill in a way that is apparently unrelated to individual survival? Reading Cartwright's book, the reader will undoubtedly feel closer to an answer to this complex puzzle.

Peter Fonagy

Acknowledgments

I am grateful to Arthur Hyatt-Williams for his useful commentary on some of the ideas put forward in this book. Much gratitude is also expressed to Rosine Perelberg, Barrie Biven, The Anna Freud Centre and the late Mervin Glasser for sending me reprints of papers I had difficulty gaining access to.

I would like to thank all prisoners at Durban Prison, South Africa, who consented to participating in the research programme. Kathija Bhamjee, senior psychologist at Durban Prison, is also thanked for her assistance with the programme. Much gratitude is expressed to those patients whom I have treated for rage-related offences and who, in doing so, have greatly informed my ideas in this area.

Some sections of this book contain revised extracts of papers published elsewhere. They appear with permission: 'The narcissistic exoskeleton: notes on the defensive organization of the rage-type murderer', *Bulletin of the Menninger Clinic*, 66(1), 1–18. Copyright © Guilford Press, 2002. 'The role of psychopathology and personality in rage-type homicide: a review', *South African Journal of Psychology*, 31: 12–19. Copyright © Psychological Society of South Africa, 2001. 'Seven intrapsychic dimensions of violence', *Psycho-analytic Psychotherapy in South Africa*, 20(1), 25–58.

Introduction

> Murder, despite our reluctance to admit it, is part of our humanity because it is rooted in human emotions.
>
> (Abrahamsen, 1973, p. 9)

A number of difficulties confront us when attempting to investigate extreme cases of violence. The acts themselves often resist any rational explanation and evoke in us a sense of fear and helplessness. To read about women or even babies being raped, family murders, sadistic killings, and other shows of violence, puts most of us through a painful process of having to think the unthinkable. Our reactions here, of course, have a lot to do with empathy for the victims of violence. It is also, however, a response that resonates with the offender's intention: to act *on*, and expel, unbearable states of mind. Through leaving his mark on the physical world, the offender also imparts in our minds the essence of what violence is about. Whether these states of mind undergo some form of perverse transformation or are controlled through a complex system of defences, whether violence is precipitated through shame or guilt, or is intended to cause suffering, at their core, all types of violence are about the expression of unbearable states of mind.

As Abrahamsen suggests, in the above brief statement, the difficulties we have in investigating extreme cases of violence are often related to how unbearable thoughts of violence or murder are generally dealt with. The way we understand and explain violence frequently reflects an avoidance of what is potentially a part of all of us. Wertham (1962), a pioneer in the field, isolates three trends that have obscured a fuller understanding of the problem. First, violence is often mystified or veiled in an intrigue that detracts from the reality of the situation. The manner in which violence is glamorized in the media or in popular culture might be understood in this way. Second, human destructiveness is often construed as 'evil', giving rise to beliefs that place it beyond the reach of scientific scrutiny. Whether glamorized or seen as evil, violence essentially becomes de-humanized, leaving us secure in the belief that it has nothing to do with the human condition.

Wertham's third observation refers to the common assumption that all murderers must suffer from extreme pathological conditions: psychosis, psychopathy, or some other form of 'mental disturbance'. The idea that acts of violence and murder are often committed by individuals who cannot easily be separated from the average man-in-the-street is far more difficult to contemplate. This is not just a lay perception. The illusion of explanation and cause that a 'scientific' diagnosis creates in the field of psychiatry is often viewed as sufficient in explaining motivations for violence. The fact that most of our dealings with murderers and serious violent offenders occur within the context of a forensic investigation does not make this any easier. The judicial system demands that the clinician produces scientific observable 'facts' about the offender that are often reduced to a psychiatric diagnosis. There is little time for understanding the underlying, and perhaps less tangible, complexities of each case here. This approach has often led to violent offenders being treated as a homogenous group, creating the impression that all murderers are the same. Homicides are grouped together simply because they have the same endpoint, that of killing.

Perhaps it is the need for observable 'facts', along with the aspiration to predict violence through 'objective' means, that has led to there being very little emphasis on understanding the role of intrapsychic factors in the development of violence. The intrapsychic world of the individual is essentially psychic reality made up of representations, drives, images, defences and mental objects; a world that makes up the subject matter of psychoanalytic inquiry. There are, I believe, many important observations to be made here to which we do not have access through 'objective' assessments of dangerousness or through the application of simple diagnostic categories. As clinicians, psychotherapists and psychoanalytic researchers we have privileged access to the internal world of others. Our insights in this regard have important implications for understanding the precipitants of extreme forms of violence, alerting us to factors that may help prevent or anticipate such acts. Without an adequate grasp of the offender's psychic reality we are unable to fully understand treatment and prognostic considerations, or to assess accurately the propensity to commit violence.

Recently there appears to have been a burgeoning interest in the study of violence in psychoanalytic circles. Authors such as Shengold, Fonagy and colleagues, Glasser, Gilligan, Perelberg, Meloy, Zulueta, to name a few, have been instrumental in making significant contributions to our understanding of violence. Developments in this area are perhaps best reflected in Perelberg's (1999a) outstanding selection of papers presented in *Psychoanalytic Understanding of Violence and Suicide*. Her review of the literature clearly shows how diverse psychoanalytic opinion is on issues related to aggression and violence. One of the key problems we face here, as Perelberg points out, arises from the confusing use of terminology. Aggression, for instance, is often used to describe a vast array of behaviours, from self-affirming practices to extreme acts of violence. Further, terms like 'aggression' and 'violence' are also regularly used to describe the intrapsychic life of the individual and often have very little to do with *actual* physical acts of violence. This leads to considerable theoretical confusion for anyone wanting to understand the origins of particular forms of aggression or violence.

In the first part of this book, Aggression and Violence in Psychoanalysis, I take up this problem. The first chapter explores the way the concept of aggression has been used in psychoanalysis. I argue that, although the models considered make some contribution to our understanding, most lack clarity in distinguishing between different forms of aggression and violence. Because of this, the inevitable differences in the psychodynamic origins of specific behavioural manifestations of aggression still remain unclear. I also suggest that the dichotomy in the debate around the instinctual and reactive origins of aggression has prevented further clarity in this regard by perpetuating the idea that aggression has only one origin. For the purposes of my investigation of rage-type murder I go on to clarify my understanding of the terms *rage* and *violence*. Here, I am in agreement with a number of authors who see violence as essentially defined by the physical act and its destructive intention, conscious or unconscious.

Violence, perhaps more than anything, has a tangible, physical end that emphatically imprints itself on external reality. As a result it demands more from our theoretical musings about the intrapsychic world, forcing us to bring the relationship between psychic reality and external reality into full focus. In this way, just as much as I intend to consider the intrapsychic aspects of rage-type murder, external reality will always be evident in the background.

With this in mind, the second chapter explores possible intrapsychic factors that translate into physical violence. Here, I review more recent psychoanalytic developments and restrict myself mostly to those who consider the *act* of violence, as opposed to those who use it more broadly as a psychological construct. Much of the work I concentrate on is drawn from an object relations perspective. My aim here is to develop a template of intrapsychic dimensions that could be used to explore different kinds of violence and, for my purpose, it lays a foundation for my investigation of rage-type murder. I argue that dimensions like representational capacity, fantasy and the quality of object relations shift in particular ways, and have varying significance, depending on the type of violence considered.

Despite there being renewed interest in understanding violence in general, comprehensive psychoanalytically-oriented studies on specific forms of violence, like particular kinds of murder, still remain limited. Exceptions here, related to the study of murder, can be found in the recent work of authors such as Meloy, Hyatt-Williams and Gilligan. But for the most, it is often difficult to discern what kind of violence is being referred to, again implying that violence is a homogenous phenomenon. This has important implications given that various forms of violence appear to have very different psychodynamic pathways.

There appears to be a number of related reasons why systematic studies on particular types of violence have been limited in psychoanalysis. I refer here particularly to the study of murder, but these reasons also apply to other forms of violence. First, psychoanalysis is often viewed as predominantly a method of treatment where research is confined to the parameters of the therapeutic setting. Therefore, unless one is in a forensic setting treating homicide offenders, research opportunities are extremely limited. Second, and related to this, psychoanalysis has been relatively slow in developing other methodologies in applied and empirical areas that would facilitate other forms of research to substantiate its claims. In short, psychoanalysis presents itself as having limited use in engaging with other forms of applied research. Unfortunately this is one of the reasons why psychoanalysis is often viewed as being isolated from other academic disciplines (Emde and Fonagy, 1997; Kirshner, 1998; Schachter and Luborsky, 1998). I am referring here particularly to the disciplines of psychiatry, psychology and criminology. Finally, the fact that the study of murder is most readily associated with the discipline of criminology also appears to discourage psychoanalytic research. Here, situational, behavioural and cognitive theoretical models are more readily adopted to suit the demands of the judicial and legal process.

Although the latter is largely the case, this is not a reason to view criminological or psychological research as contrary to the psychoanalytic cause. Actuarial details of violence and murder used in criminological, psychological and psychiatric research can be useful in verifying analytic insights and can also help define areas of interest that require exploration from a psychoanalytic point of view. In keeping with this, although I intend to address the problem of violence from a psychoanalytic perspective, I have drawn on other sources of research where I have found it necessary to develop my argument.

RAGE-TYPE MURDER

With these general theoretical issues discussed, the rest of this volume investigates rage-type murder as a specific form of violence. I use the term to refer to murder that has been motivated primarily by explosive rage. Although often provoked, such acts appear senseless and motiveless, with the offender displaying a degree of dissociation during the event.

I include here three brief examples of rage-type murder that have made headlines in the press during my writing of this introduction. In the first, a man on his way home from work became enraged with another motorist who had accidentally cut in front of him. He managed to stop his victim and after a brief exchange of insults, bludgeoned him to death with a hockey stick. The victim's skull bore the signs of repeated powerful blows to the head. In another incident, a loving father of two repeatedly stabbed his wife to death with a kitchen knife after she had refused his embrace. The report claims that the couple had decided to separate a week prior to the murder. In a final example, a successful businessman turned his gun on his family after a quarrel with his wife. He shot all but one of his family members in a spray of bullets and then attempted to turn the gun on himself.

In all the above accounts the offender was described as being 'mentally stable' with no previous history of violence. In reports searching for explanations for such aberrant behaviour we often hear a range of reasons: he was unhappy in his marriage; his wife was abusive; he had felt deeply insulted; his wife had cheated on him; he had been having a difficult time at work. All these, of course, may be valid sources of provocation, but none are enough to explain why this should lead to murder or extreme violence.

In the latter example, the man who killed most of his family, the offender's brother and a work colleague were interviewed after the crime and described him as 'a perfectionist who took great pride in his work', 'a man who has extremely high morals and standards, an example to others', 'a successful leader of his firm who treated his employees like family and would do anything for others'.

How should we make sense of such statements? Claims like this are typical and often form part of an attempt to come to terms with the extreme dissonance between the offender's general character and the aberrant act of violence. Certainly, such claims could be understood as a simple consequence of relativity and polarization where, relative to an act of murder, all other behaviours are perceived as quite 'normal' and may even be seen as fine examples of 'good' behaviour. Notwithstanding this however, in my view, such statements also reflect a degree of truth in portraying the offender's general approach and personality. Much of what is to come in this book is essentially an attempt to identify and understand intrapsychic factors that give rise to what I understand to be an over-controlled and encapsulated personality.

To this end, the two remaining parts of this book set out to explore the internal world of those who have committed acts of murder similar to those described above. I am essentially concerned with questions about what it means, at an intrapsychic level, to commit an act of murder. More precisely, I am concerned with understanding what it means to commit murder *in this way*. It should be pointed out that I am not making the claim that a single personality type or psychodynamic profile can account for all acts of explosive violence. Clearly, a broad spectrum of individuals are capable of such acts, from severely disturbed psychotic patients to hardened serial offenders; all have different motivations for violence. I am interested in a particular group of offenders who have rigid, encapsulated personalities that make them vulnerable to rare, but extremely damaging, shows of violence.

In the first chapter in this section the clinical features and parameters of the act are explored. Following this I broaden my investigation to explore dilemmas regarding personality and the presence of psychopathology in such individuals. Here I draw on contributions from psychiatry, psychology and criminology. One of the key points of discussion in this chapter is the apparent normality of rage-type offenders. These kinds of offender are not usually violent, show few signs of psychopathology and do not have psychopathic motives for committing murder. Their aberrant rage is thus far more difficult to understand. The overcontrolling nature of the personality and its encapsulated character appears to shed some light on the problem and it is suggested that these characteristics appear to describe an atypical borderline personality organization. In the final chapter of this section I explore a number of seminal psychodynamic studies on murder raising a variety of questions to be pursued in later chapters.

The final section is devoted to considering the intrapsychic dimensions of rage-type murder using the dimensions developed earlier. Most notably, a specific kind of defensive organization is apparent in these offenders. I term the defensive organization the 'narcissistic exoskeleton' and devote a chapter to exploring its function in relation to explosive violence and the apparent stability of the personality. It is characterized by a particular kind of splitting that strives to keep an internalized bad object system separate from idealized good objects. The idealized object system itself appears to serve a defensive function here and requires constant attention to ensure that bad objects, associated with aggression, remain unarticulated and split-off in the psyche.

Other factors such as poor representational capacity, the absence of violent fantasy, the absence of a clearly defined paternal object, and the way particular situational factors impinge on the individual are discussed as significant features of the offender's psychological make-up. Following this, I return to the act itself to consolidate my understanding of how minor provocations may have led to murder in cases explored. A reconstruction of the probable dynamic sequence of events is presented and it appears that the collapse of narcissistic defences, exposure to unbearable shame, and the use of evacuative projective identifications best explain this process. In the final chapter, I consider some ideas related to assessment, psychotherapy and prevention.

Although my observations yield various intrapsychic factors that appear prominent in the rage-type offender, I am not suggesting that such individuals are 'programmed' to eventually commit murder. This may be accurate for some killers who are driven by powerful urges to act out violent fantasy. The situation, however, is usually more complex. In my view, unless particular intrapsychic factors and external reality come together in a particular way, at a particular point in time, murder will not take place. In other words, I am not suggesting that individuals who display a similar defensive organization to the one outlined later, will eventually commit murder. The act is dependent on a number of factors or dimensions. They are best understood as being vulnerability factors that may not always lead to violence. I hope to show, however, in my analysis of those who have killed, that preparation for murder begins long before the act itself.

Part I

Aggression and violence in psychoanalysis

Chapter 1

Aggression, rage and violence

> No one questions the experiential evocation of aggression – aggression as a response to frustration, deprivation, pain, overstimulation. What we do not know is whether it starts from within as an innate drive or as a reaction to something without.
>
> (Shengold, 1999, p.xiii)

The term *aggression* is often used in very broad and confusing ways in psycho-analytic literature. Much of the confusion comes from the use of the term to refer to both a psychological drive and/or a behavioural action. Perelberg (1999a) defines aggression as 'a variety of behaviours, feelings, and representations, from attempts to master the environment to something that is perceived as destructive' (p. 40). Aggression is thus seen as having constructive and destructive aims. Whilst some have emphasized both its neutralized constructive potential as well as its harmful nature, others argue that aggression is distinctly destructive and should be separated from positive terms such as assertiveness and psychic activity. The above distinctions are all ultimately derived from what one understands the nature of aggression to be. This, of course, remains a perennial debate in psychoanalysis stretched between those who view it as reactive in nature and those who view it as instinctual.

I shall begin by reviewing Freud's understanding of aggression and then go on to consider both sides of the debate, highlighting some of the main theories and contributions on the nature of aggression. The emphasis here is on considering how aggression as an intrapsychic occurrence has been formulated. In particular, the status of the internal object within these formulations will be considered. Although regarded by some as simply an intellectual debate, this has important implications for how we understand, treat and make prognostic assumptions about pathological states.

I shall argue that even in Freud's work, the many different ways in which aggression is understood hints at a problem that the nature–nurture debate on aggression has obscured from full view. Whilst the debate is of great importance, with both sides shedding light on different aspects of aggression, it draws us into the spurious position of believing that there is one kind of aggression that must have one origin.

With this argument in place, I briefly consider the concept of rage as a particular form of aggression with specific psychological determinants. Finally, the broad features of what constitutes violent action are explored. The definitions of violence outlined here bear testimony to the complex origins of different forms of aggression.

THE NATURE AND OBJECT OF AGGRESSION

Freud on aggression

It is often argued that Freud only considered aggression to be an important component of the personality when he began to formulate the nature of aggression as being linked to the death instinct (Freud, 1920). His ideas on aggression, however, were far more complex than being simply about the externalization of the death instinct.

Freud first briefly mentions the role of aggression in 'Three essays on the theory of sexuality' (1905a) and 'Fragment of an analysis of a case of hysteria' (1905b). In the former he finds aggression to be a means of sexual mastery over an object. In the latter he considers it a form of resistance to treatment. His first comprehensive attempt to understand aggression, however, can be found in 'Instincts and their vicissitudes' (Freud, 1915). In this paper he explores elements of love and hate and their relation to self-preservative and sexual instincts.

Freud argues that, during the pre-genital stages of development love and hate are indistinguishable and the infant remains indifferent to his own sadistic actions and injury to his objects. The primary motive at this stage, through incorporating and devouring the object, is the urge for mastery over the object. However, he argues that hate itself has a different instinctual source based in the self-preservative instincts:

> The ego hates, abhors and pursues with intent to destroy all objects which are the source of unpleasurable feeling for it, without taking into account whether they mean a frustration of sexual satisfaction or the satisfaction of self-preservative needs. Indeed it may be asserted that the true prototypes of the relation of hate are derived not from sexual life, but from the ego's struggle to preserve and maintain itself.
>
> (Freud, 1915, p.136)

It is only later on in development that sadism proper emerges when sadistic tendencies are internalized and fused with the sexual instincts to form masochistic object relations. In turn, when this is externalized again, aggressive tendencies have become associated with pleasure, and the pain inflicted on the object begins to accrue a sexual motive. The external object, when first presented, is hated and seen as a source of unpleasure because it challenges the individual's narcissistic conception of the world. Freud describes the genesis of hate as follows:

> Hate, as a relation to objects, is older than love. It derives from the narcissistic ego's primordial repudiation of the external world with its outpouring of stimuli. As an expression of the reaction of unpleasure evoked by objects, it always remains in an intimate relation with the self-preservative instincts.
>
> (Freud, 1915, p.135)

With the introduction of the death instinct in 'Beyond the pleasure principle' (1920), Freud's understanding of aggression took a new turn. Aggression was now seen as an innate manifestation of the death drive, although not simply equated with the death instinct. Here, he reserves the term aggression for the externalization of the death instinct.

Freud's need to postulate the existence of the death instinct did not come directly from a need to explain the expression of aggressiveness. He sought primarily to understand how the repetition of unpleasant phenomena in the form of the repetition compulsion did not abide by the pleasure principle. Using evidence from the biological sciences he concludes his speculation with the observation that all living organisms hold within them the seeds of their own destruction: an element of instinctual life that seeks to return living matter to an inanimate state. Apart from aggression having a different function here, sadism is now seen as being secondary to masochistic dynamics. The death instinct seeks its own form of satisfaction characterized by internal pain.

Still later, in terms of his structural model, Freud begins to view unconscious guilt as the result of 'a piece of aggressiveness that has been internalized and taken over by the superego' (Freud, 1933, p.142). He describes the superego as being, in part, a construction made up of aggression that has been taken in from the outside world. There is no sign of the death instinct here at first. But Freud goes on to suggest that the superego may also absorb aspects of the 'destructive instinct' (p.143) that could not be discharged onto external objects: 'aggressiveness may not be able to find satisfaction in the external world because it comes up against real obstacles. If this happens it will perhaps retreat and increase the amount of self-destructiveness holding sway in the interior.' (Freud, 1933, p.138).

Freud claims that the relative harshness of the superego, observed in neurotics, compared to lower levels of strictness and aggression found in their external world confirms the occurrence of the above process. The destructiveness of the superego thus becomes a key dynamic in understanding melancholia, neuroses and masochism (Freud, 1923).

Freud is never conclusive about the role of aggression in the personality, especially about how his earlier work on aggressiveness and hate should be considered alongside the death instinct. We may assume perhaps that the self-preservative instincts, which become part of the life instincts in his revised model, would still retain elements of aggressiveness aimed outwards in the service of the preservation of the ego. In support of this, Perelberg (1995b) points out that Freud, in 'Analysis terminable and interminable', also introduced the concept of 'free aggressiveness'. This type of aggression could attach itself to any instinct with the effect of creating the coexistence of contradictory affective states. It offers a possible explanation as to why the instinct of self-preservation always has some measure of aggressiveness in its action.

Often, the opposition between sexuality and aggression is confused and seen as the same as the opposition between the life and death instincts, which has tended to misrepresent Freud's understanding of aggression. Aggression cannot be accounted for as simply emanating from the destructive motives of the death drive. As Anna Freud (1972) and later Perelberg (1995b) have argued, Freud shows aggression to have different sources of development which cannot be confined to this opposition. It could be said that Freud's ideas reflect the difficulties inherent in much of the literature on aggression: although one type or source of aggression is sought, a consideration of how the term is used in many different ways, hints at a more complex problem.

In summary, Freud considered four different manifestations of aggression that may exist internally or otherwise be discharged. They are: aggression that has its roots in self-preservation and protection of the ego; free-floating aggression; aggression that emerges from the externalization of the death instinct which, by definition, has a destructive aim; and aggression that has an intrapsychic location and is absorbed by the superego and turned against the ego. Although never integrated into a single theory of aggression, both reactive and instinctual elements are evident here.

I turn now to considering subsequent arguments and theories related to considering aggression as instinct or reaction before considering the essence of the debate further. This review is far from exhaustive. Rather, I have selected a few positions that best illustrate the diverse ways in which the concept of aggression has been used.

Aggression as instinct

Hering (1997) lauds Freud's efforts in placing human destructiveness firmly within the individual through the formulation of the death instinct:

> Whatever you might think of Freud's concept of a death drive which opposes all forms of life, one has to pay tribute to his courage. Not only did he envisage a force of silent and absolute destructive intention, he also did not hesitate to place it within each man's and each woman's own psyche. By doing so he set a frame within which the struggle with this 'evil' could take place in a less externalized and alienated form.
>
> (Hering, 1997, p.211)

Although it has its supporters (for example Abraham, 1927; Hitchcock, 1996;

Klein, 1957; Segal, 1997; Shengold, 1991), the death instinct, or the idea of an aggressive drive, still remains one of the most contentious theoretical ideas put forward by Freud. Many believe that there is little need to postulate an entirely separate destructive instinct in order to understand aggression (Fromm, 1973; Glasser, 1998; Kernberg, 1980; Stern, 1985).

Zulueta (1993), a vehement opponent of the death instinct theory, views it as nothing more than a cultural construct emanating from Western Christian belief systems, particularly the belief in the original sin. To view destructiveness and wickedness as an innate component of humanity, she argues, clears the individual of personal responsibility and also helps emphasize man's inability to control himself. More importantly, she argues that the idea of the death instinct has never disappeared – despite research to the contrary – because it has become the easiest way to give meaning to suffering. It also gives us reason to feel guilty rather than simply out of control and helpless. Further, Zulueta claims that viewing love and hate as derivatives of opposite drives prevents the exploration of the links between them. As a consequence, it fails to give appropriate emphasis to the link between violence and our need for stable loving attachments.

Ornstein and Ornstein (1993) explore the clinical consequences of dual drive theory explaining that if aggression is considered to be a drive, aggression itself can no longer be analysed, only the way it is managed becomes responsive to analytic interventions. A further consequence of dual instinct theory relates to the idea that the release of aggression through the analytic process will put an end to neurotic symptoms. These theorists find it more useful, however, to focus on the need to keep aggression out of the transference in order to maintain self-cohesiveness. From a different perspective, Kernberg (1980) dismisses the Kleinian death instinct on the basis that it has no clinical significance and cannot be observed in any meaningful way. Many others have also argued that the death instinct has received little clinical substantiation (Fairbairn, 1952; Glasser, 1998; Guntrip, 1968; Kohut, 1978) and some have pointed to a lack of empirical verification regarding the concept (Hollin, 1989; Parens, 1993).

Those who have supported the concept claim that the power of the death instinct is clinically observable (Klein, 1957; Segal, 1997; Rosenfeld, 1971; Shengold, 1991) and the nature of human destructiveness cannot be simply explained as a response to frustration. Segal (1997), for instance, illustrates how feelings of dead-ness and despair in the countertransference are often projected manifestations of the death instinct. Rosenfeld (1987), on the other hand, uses his observations of 'destructive narcissism' as evidence of the death instinct. Shengold (1999) argues that transference–countertransference resistances make it difficult to deal with the idea of an aggressive drive. He thinks that this often keeps us from acknowledging and theorizing its importance:

> It is my conviction that murder, the aggressive drive to violence – central to both the preoedipal and oedipal in Freudian and Kleinian theory – has been consistently underplayed as a motivational force because it gives rise to so

much anxiety and so much resistance in clinical work, on the part of analysts as well as patients.

(Shengold, 1999, p.xv)

Although the idea of the death instinct itself is difficult to prove, one would be hard pressed to prove that aggression does not have its roots in instinct, no matter how remote. Ethological research reminds us of how difficult it is to divorce psychology entirely from biology. The protective aggressive displays that can readily be observed in the animal kingdom, for instance, cannot be fully divorced from our own behaviours (Konner, 1993; Lorenz, 1963; Schuster, 1978). One might argue that this is especially the case when we consider the disproportionate ways in which aggression is expressed across the sexes. Here, biological, genetic and basic instinctual links to aggression cannot be ignored.

It is often held that the struggle between representatives of life and death can just as easily be formulated in purely psychological terms (Brenner, 1971). What this precept lacks, however, is a link to the body. One of Freud's key motivations for considering the instinctual nature of man in understanding the psychology of the individual was to provide an essential link to the body and biological processes. I would agree with Schafer (1976) in arguing that the physiological characteristics of aggression and its 'bodily' nature are often underestimated by non-drive theorists. He views aggression as a 'psychophysiological reaction' which occurs in a relational context rather than simply being seen as an isolated spontaneous bodily impulse. Similarly, Kernberg (1984) sees the rejection of the instinctual nature of aggression as disregarding the biological forerunners of human development. Given that the nature of the link between aggression and the body is the essence of what constitutes a violent act, biological variants, such as instinctual and neurophysiological make-up, are difficult to ignore.

Ideas pertaining to the instinctual nature of aggression have been developed in two main directions since Freud. These directions are most evident in the *Kleinian* and *Ego Psychology* schools, the former being the principal advocate of the death instinct. They both provide possible explanations for how the origins of aggression can be formulated intrapsychically.

Klein (1932) bases much of her psychological understanding of the individual on Freud's ideas of the death instinct. Based on clinical observations with children, she argued that envy and destructiveness dominate in early life as derivatives of the death instinct and are responsible for primary forms of anxiety in the psyche. Through projective and introjective mechanisms the infant's main task at this very early stage is to split off all part-objects that have become 'bad' through their association with destructiveness which, in turn, results in further paranoid anxiety (Klein, 1946). Klein found the death instinct to be a useful concept for explaining what she observed to be a much earlier formation of an archaic harsh superego (Klein, 1928). For her, the formation of this primitive internalized object resulted from the internalization of the death instinct that had initially been projected outwards onto other objects.

Central to the Kleinian approach is the observation that phantasies, the psychic derivatives of the life and death instincts, are always object related (Isaacs, 1948; Klein, 1958). There is no such thing as primary narcissism or a destructive object-less state. The central implication of this for understanding aggression is that Kleinian formulations are not driven by energetic or homeostatic principles where discharge is the essential driving force, placing the significance of the object as secondary. Klein began from the premise that the object is always present in phantasy constellations, setting up an object-related dynamic from which aggression emanates. Her concept of projective identification also shifted the meaning of aggressiveness from simply being a deflection of the death instinct away from the self (Freud, 1920) to a more complex understanding of destructiveness. Because projective identification always involves a part of the self, aggression is 'directed both at the perceiving self and the object perceived' (Segal, 1997, p.18). Thus, the deflection or projection of aggression also has important consequences for the self. First, parts of the self are also attacked in this process in their projected state. Second, projection identification leads to further depletion of the self.

Later, Bion (1970) developed this central idea by postulating a *container–contained relationship* as a key theoretical configuration that, amongst other things, existed between mother and infant. His work allowed for a more developed understanding of how the maternal function works to metabolize innate destructive aspects of the infant's psyche through projective and introjective processes. His work also developed Klein's ideas on evacuative forms of projective identification that play a key role in understanding aggressive responses intrapsychically and interpersonally.

The work of innate destructiveness still remains central to understanding pathological states in Kleinian circles (for example Bateman, 1999; Grotstein, 1981; Rosenfeld, 1987; Segal, 1991; Spillius, 1988; Steiner, 1993). For this reason this body of work is perhaps the most systematic study of the role of destructiveness in character development. It would be wrong to assume, however, that the Kleinian perspective largely excludes positive life-giving forces evident in the psyche, as some have argued (Greenberg and Mitchell, 1983; Chessick, 1993). Indeed, much of Klein's own later work, most evident in 'Envy and Gratitude' (Klein, 1957) is an attempt to understand creative forces in the psyche.

The other main development in conceptualizing the instinctual nature of aggression comes from those who have laid primary emphasis on the development of the ego. Although retaining the dual instinct theory, Hartmann *et al.* (1949) emphasize the neutralizing function of the ego that serves to 'deinstinctualize' both sexual and aggressive instincts, in turn, lessening their need for discharge. Neutralization differs from Freud's idea of sublimation in that it is not a defence against drive demand, nor is it a deflection onto another object. It represents a transformation process that is an important part of psychic development.

In this way Hartmann conceptualizes the structural components of the psyche as made up of different energy systems ultimately derived from both the sexual and aggressive drives. He also argues, however, that the ego has, in addition, its own innate adaptive features that come from other forms of psychic energy, although he is never clear on this issue (Greenberg and Mitchell, 1983). For Hartmann, the internalization of object relations has an important influence on determining the aggressive nature of the individual. The infant interacts with an 'average expectable environment' that ensures the appropriate neutralization of the drives. However, Hartmann clearly rejects theorists who see the role of the internalized object as having a direct influence on the individual. He is loyal to Freud in this regard, seeing all interaction as being mediated through the drives first. Nevertheless, later authors, particularly Jacobson (1954) followed by Kernberg (1966), have modified this view claiming that the bifurcation of the drives is directly dependent on the nature of objects that are internalized. In other words, inchoate object relations have a primary influence on how the drives become polarized.

To return to Hartmann, aggression here is primarily determined by an innate aggressive charge and the neutralizing function of the ego. Hartmann takes issue with Freud's claims that the aggressive drive does not follow the pleasure principle. According to him, the suppression of all psychic drives leads to increased unpleasure, whilst drive expression leads to pleasure. He further believes that the ego has a degree of autonomy in determining what will be pleasurable and what will be unpleasurable.

The repetition compulsion thus becomes reformulated as no longer a manifestation of the death instinct *per se*, but is accounted for by the need to act on pleasure-filled activity. Brenner (1971) points out that this appears to have been accepted by most psychoanalysts but it has not been followed by the relevant theory to back it up. It is not clear, for instance, whether this kind of 'pleasure' is not better termed 'relief' in the sense that it is linked directly to the release of an unbearable psychic state that differs from libidinal satisfaction.

If emphasis is placed on the ego, the aim of aggression depends largely on ego strength and how defence mechanisms manage the developmental process. If appropriate neutralization takes place, aggression can be used in the service of the ego, emerging in acts or states of assertiveness to further personal growth. The positive use of aggression for self-assertion and the establishment of boundaries between self and other is also a common feature of many of the reactive models of aggression.

Destructive aggression, on the other hand, occurs when the ego is weak. From this point of view, a person may have murderous or aggressive tendencies, but whether these are acted out or not depends on the strength of the ego. Importantly, however, the ego can also be over-cathected leading to rigid ego–id boundaries where repression becomes restrictive and where none of the aggressive or libidinal drives can be sublimated and the person's affective range remains shallow and ineffective (Kutash, 1978).

In sum then, viewing aggression as a drive to be neutralized and used positively in the psyche holds up a far more optimistic view of the individual's struggle with aggression. Viewing aggression as more directly entrenched in the death instinct, on the other hand, immediately places the individual in a hateful world. Here, hate and dread are central to primitive experience and it is only if these can be contained in some way, that love and the 'good object' can be found. Furthermore, according to the Kleinian approach, this level of primitive experience will always exist embedded deep in phantasy, constantly influencing our everyday experience. Viewing the individual as being aggressive by nature is very different from considering the origins of aggression as rooted in reaction or interaction.

Aggression as reaction

Those who have rejected the notion of innate destructiveness, or the presence of an aggressive drive, tend to agree broadly on conceptualizing aggression as a reaction to frustration, unpleasure, or threat from an internal/external object. Fairbairn (1952), Guntrip (1968), Kohut (1972), and Parens (1993), to name a few, all clearly advocate this view using different theoretical means. There is a focus here on the deprivation of need being related to destructive aggression, something that Freud was unable to separate from the frustration of instinct (Gallwey, 1985). Specific emphasis has also been placed on reaction to loss, trauma and difficulties with attachments (Bowlby, 1969; Hyatt-Williams, 1998; Zulueta, 1993). Here, the defensive nature of aggression, as a means of protection and warding off threat, is emphasized.

The key factor that underlies all reactive models is the emphasis on the role of the object, primarily the maternal object, in the development of aggressiveness itself. This approach to understanding aggression is perhaps best exemplified in the work of Winnicott and Fairbairn to which I shall now turn. Winnicott's emphasis is placed on the role of the maternal environment, whilst Fairbairn focuses on understanding manifestations of aggression in complex internal object constellations.

Whilst not rejecting the idea of instinct *per se*, Winnicott (1971) preferred to conceptualize instinct as a spontaneous, creative force. The origins of aggression could be found in the earliest forms of infantile bodily movement equivalent to all bodily activity at this stage. Aggression here is viewed as a positive force that allows the infant, through spontaneous motoric movements, to discover his or her own limitations. In his terms, it allows the infant to discover the difference between what is 'me' and 'not me' and serves as the primary means for establishing 'object permanence'.

The steps for maternal environmental provision and the course of 'normal' aggressiveness are as follows: First, initial ego-support allows for an element of 'destruction by chance' emanating from the infant's exploration of the environment with little impingement from reality. The 'good-enough' mother then gradually goes through a process of disillusionment, allowing the introduction of reality and a reduction of magical qualities attached to what is omnipotently controlled and aggressed by the infant. Finally, the actual survival of the mother, unchanged, when she has been 'destroyed', or placed outside the infant's subjective self, creates a stable permanent object relationship. The mother 'survives' the attacks and importantly, has not retaliated.

Winnicott (1986) believed that 'the antisocial tendency', which included a broad range of negative behaviours including destructive aggression, was directly linked to deprivation, as opposed to privation. He believed that these individuals had once 'known' a good-enough mother and thus had felt some sense of ego-support and integration, but this had been lost. At that point the child suffers 'unthinkable anxiety' and then is 'gradually reorganized into someone who is in a fairly neutral state, complying because there is nothing else that the child is strong enough to do' (p.92). Although Winnicott does not link this to the origins of the False Self in his work, the state of compliance described here appears very similar to what he describes as the False Self in other publications (Winnicott, 1965).

Antisocial behaviour, as he understood it, was about attempting to 'get back behind the deprivation moment ... to undo the unthinkable anxiety or confusion that resulted before the neutral state became organized' (Winnicott, 1986, p.92). It marks the rediscovery of aggressiveness and at the same time, a moment of hope. Aggressiveness here expresses the attitude 'the environment owes me something' (Winnicott, 1965, p.134), an expression of wanting what he or she once had. In other words, for Winnicott, destructiveness is never an end in itself and in this way is similar to Self Psychology's perspective on aggression (Kohut, 1978; Chessick, 1993). It is the point at which the individual has the 'courage' to put the False Self aside and allow the True Self to express itself. This idea has been used in a number of different ways to understand violent behaviour, to which we shall return later.

Fairbairn (1952) also believed that destructive aggression had its roots in deprivation. Concentrating less on the role of the mother *per se*, he set out to understand the kind of intrapsychic structural dynamics that deprivation set up. In doing so, he formulated a model of the personality that represents the most radical shift away from Freudian drive psychology. Central to his model is the assumption that libidinal and aggressive elements of the psyche are primarily object seeking as opposed to being pleasure or unpleasure seeking.

Fairbairn's conceptualization of aggression begins with the internalization of a rejecting maternal object. The rejecting experience sets up a central ambivalent dilemma where if 'he expresses aggression, he is threatened with the loss of his good object, and, if, on the other hand, he expresses libidinal need, he is threatened with the loss of his libido (which for him constitutes his own goodness) and ultimately the loss of the ego structure which constitutes himself' (p.113). Fairbairn found that the key solution to this dilemma took place through the internalization of the bad-mother-object in order to control it internally.

This moment leads to the complex formation of an internalized system of object relationships in which aggression plays a key role: the internalized bad object undergoes a further split into the needed or *exciting object*, and the *rejecting object*. Aggression, at this point, is used internally in two ways. It first serves the purpose of repressing these bad internalized objects. Second, a further 'volume', as Fairbairn puts it, of aggression is used to effect corresponding splits in the central ego to form subsidiary egos (the libidinal ego and the internal saboteur). These, in turn, attach themselves to their corresponding split-off parts of the internalized object.

With this internal structure in place, aggressive affect is absorbed by the internal saboteur and used to attack any needs that the libidinal ego may have towards its external object. In Fairbairn's terms:

> The child seeks to circumvent the dangers of expressing both libidinal and aggressive affect towards his object by using a maximum of his aggression to subdue a maximum of libidinal need. In this way he reduces the volume of affect, both libidinal and aggressive, demanding outward expression.
>
> (Fairbairn, 1952, pp.114–15)

The child's aggressive feelings towards mother thus live on in an internalized situation where aggression is turned on a repressed part of the self with the effect of destroying libidinal need.

Apart from being the 'purest' attempt to understand human motivations from a psychological, as opposed to a biological perspective, Fairbairn's approach is an attempt to trace the internal object relationships that lie behind aggression. In essence his approach is based on the individual's attempt to control bad objects through internalization. Aggression has two main functions: First, it functions to repress the bad object that has been split in two. Second, it is used to launch an internal attack on the libidinal, needy parts of the subsidiary ego.

The idea that aggression may be reactive is beyond debate to most. Whether it is originally so is more difficult to ascertain. With their differences in emphasis, the importance of Winnicott's and Fairbairn's approaches lies in their ability to demonstrate the possible origins of aggression through interaction and object relationships. For them, aggression originates between objects and is not simply an innate destructive force that uses the object as a vehicle for discharge.

BEYOND THE DEBATE: ONE AGGRESSION OR MANY?

Thus far we have considered some of the main approaches and problems associated with understanding aggression. All these approaches have value in their own right. But how then does one ascertain which view to follow? Is it simply a matter of how one chooses to understand the human condition as Perelberg (1999a) attests. Or does it depend on the type of behaviour, emotion and so forth being observed?

Taking the latter view, I would argue that the polarization that has occurred between different theories is the result of asking the wrong questions. Although many of the theories discussed above side with one end of the debate, do we need to conclude that there is only one answer? Implicit in many of the writings on aggression are references to different types, functions and aims allocated to what is broadly termed 'aggression'. I think that the need to see aggression as *either* instinct or reaction, nature or nurture, and as one entity, has under-emphasized specific questions regarding the nature and function of aggression/s.

A number of authors have concluded that the instinctual and reaction models of aggression need not be viewed as incompatible (Fonagy *et al.*, 1993a; Glasser, 1998; Mitchell, 1993; Shengold, 1999). Some have argued that the compatibility of these ideas is often implicit in the literature. However, this is seldom clearly stated or explored because traditional metapsychological theory cannot cope with these oppositions, indicating that some re-formulation is required.

Mitchell (1993) has attempted to show how these two apparently polarized views may be preserved within a single theory of aggression. He argues that if aggression is considered within a relational context which explores the conditions that elicit aggression, particularly what the individual brings to the interpersonal field, the instinctual and relational nature of aggression can be considered together. In his words, 'to characterize aggression as a response does not minimize its biological basis; rather, the biology of aggression is understood to operate not as a drive but as an individually constituted, pre-wired potential that is evoked by circumstances perceived as threatening or endangering' (p.364). In other words, he considers the capacity for aggression to be innate, but the aggressive happening itself is initiated by a reaction that the endangered self might experience in relation to external or internal objects.

There are many other ways of formulating the instinctual and reactive nature of aggression in one theory. It is only Symington (1996) who boldly rejects both models in favour of a model based on unconscious murderous guilt. Glasser (1998) fully acknowledges the role of the external environment in aggressive responses but argues that this does not mean that innate predispositions do not have a role to play in structuring these responses. In his words, 'aggression/violence and the stimuli that prompt it are artificially separated components of a unity: the triggers can only be regarded as such in the context of the innate structure' (Glasser, 1998, p.890). Taking a different position, Gaddini (1992) argues that frustration itself can be understood as a manifestation of instinct. Shengold (1991), on the other hand, takes the middle ground claiming that frustration, and consequent aggression, should be seen as both a reaction to the difficult demands of the environment and a response to the threat that innate destructiveness can cause.

On reviewing Freud's understanding of aggression earlier, I suggested that he points to different manifestations of aggression that cannot all just be reduced to the work of the death instinct. In other words, Freud himself appears to have struggled with this problem and, although aggression is fundamentally perceived to be instinctual in nature, he does consider the role of the object in triggering aggression, both intrapsychically and interpersonally. Freud's initial attempts thus reflect some of the difficulties that have continually been evident in this area of study.

It appears to me that attempts to build a broad theory of aggression that does not seek to simply find instinct or reaction as primary causes, better suits our needs in exploring a broad range of aggressive phenomena. Building coherent and flexible theory, however, is only part of the problem. We first need to avoid thinking about aggression as a static construct that always has the same origin and composition.

Since Freud, aggression has become reified as a single construct leading to the illusion that there is a single solution, a single way in which instinct and/or reaction make up the aggressive response. Perhaps there are many reasons for this. One of the main reasons, however, appears to stem from a quest in psychoanalysis to remain scientifically credible by succumbing to the confused belief that there can be only one scientifically correct answer, one cause and one effect. Ironically this has lead to an unfocused diffuseness in the debate where terms are often used very differently and the kind of aggression being referred to often lacks a specific reference point in 'objective' behaviours, affects, thoughts and so forth.

Although, broadly speaking, aggression may be both reactive and instinctual, the debate has obscured real questions about specific factors that may play a particular role in different forms of aggression. Put another way, 'aggression' does not have to come from the same place, intrapsychically or otherwise. Person (1993a) takes up this point arguing for the need for new models to account for the diversity of phenomena evident in aggression, rage and anger. 'Even if an aggressive drive in humans were demonstrated,' she claims,

> it would be erroneous to attribute to it all of the various manifestations of aggression, rage and anger – just as when we talk about sex, it would be extremely naive to attribute all manifestations of sexuality to the sex drive.
>
> (p.6)

A number of other researchers who have applied their minds to specific forms of violence and aggression appear to have moved beyond this debate with this realization in mind (Duncan and Duncan, 1978; Fonagy and Target, 1995; Glasser, 1998; Hyatt-Williams, 1996; Kutash, 1978; Lewis, 1993; Meloy and Gacono, 1992; Mitchell, 1993; Mullen and Maack, 1985; Parens 1993; Person, 1993a; Shengold, 1991).

All these authors acknowledge that the analysis of different forms of aggression is dependent on the relational field from which the behaviours emanate. This could be about both intrapsychic and external relations. The specifics of the situation are where a more refined understanding of aggressive phenomena lies, enabling us to understand whether we are indeed talking about the same thing. Those who have explored the specific internal and external situations linked to aggression have, I believe, been able to make a more decisive contribution to understanding aggression. Rage, violence, violence towards inanimate objects, anger, passive-aggressiveness, self-destructiveness, assertiveness and so forth – all have different psychological, psychodynamic, social and even biological correlates and influences that require separate study.

Assertiveness, for instance, may be seen as having distinctly separate influences as compared to destructive aggression (Meyers, 1993; Ornstein and Ornstein, 1993; Person, 1993a). The role of affective states has also been found to differ greatly across various forms of aggressive experience. Further, Parens (1993), in his child and infant observation studies, finds support for the existence of an aggressive drive but also finds that reactive hostile destructiveness should be viewed as a separate form of aggression caused by 'excessive unpleasure' (p.123). Another example of the different influences specific to different forms of aggression can be found in Fonagy *et al.*'s (1993b) work. They find that environmental influences, particularly the maternal object, appear to be more crucial when the infant is temperamentally difficult.

Rage can also be separated, both phenomenologically and dynamically, from other forms of aggression (Kernberg, 1992; Lewis, 1993; Person, 1993a; Symington, 1996; Treurniet, 1996). Similarly, others have been able to begin to show how different forms of violence, as specific manifestations of aggression, have different origins or correlates. All the above examples suggest that general references to aggression are problematic and specific factors related to different types of aggressive experience require greater emphasis if we are accurately to understand the many different manifestations of aggressive experience. To this end, and for the purpose of further exploring the nature of aggression apparent in rage-type murder, I turn now to considering the concepts of rage and violence.

RAGE

Not unlike the lay understanding of the term, I understand rage to be the expression of a primitive explosive affective state. Although it may well be linked to violence and vice versa, the one does not necessarily imply the other. One may, for example, fly into a rage about someone cutting in front of one on the highway, without any sign of physical violence. On the other hand, a sadistic killer may commit heinous crimes of violence without feeling any emotion that approximates rage. A number of key underlying psychodynamic factors constantly emerge in the literature pertaining to rage, the most common features being its link to self-exposure, shame, narcissistic injury, hate and reactive affective states.

Parens (1993), in his infant observational study, claims to have found no evidence for the death instinct as being the source of rage. He argues that rage is experience dependent and occurs because of 'excessive unpleasure', creating an explosive affective state. The persistence of these kinds of experiences results in the emergence of hate towards the object, especially when experienced in the first year of life. As he puts it, 'When such excessive unpleasure experiences persist, occur frequently enough, and are sufficiently intense from the first year on, they stabilize into *hate*, a more enduring feeling of self-object-attached hostile destructiveness' (1993, p.127).

Because of an accumulation of past trauma, rage reactions may more easily be triggered by a stimulus of a low intensity causing excessive reactions to seemingly benign events. In a similar way it is likely that those who have experienced recent severe trauma will also have a greatly reduced capacity for containing feelings of rage, shame and humiliation. Whether this always translates into violent action will be considered elsewhere. However, intensity, duration and frequency of unpleasure experiences also appear to determine the intensity of the rage reaction and the cumulative effects it has on the self.

Although always a reaction, the response is often understood as being an automatic involuntary reflex similar to that observed in the animal kingdom and often referred to as the *fight–flight response* to a threat (Konner, 1993). The impact that rage and its precipitants have on a human life, however, is where we differ from animals. We are able to remember, *re-present* and think about threats and dangers. They do not simply go away after cathartic discharge, or, in time, lead to simple learned responses, as they do with animals. *They linger on and have a psychic life.* The internalization of such dangers has varied consequences. If such dangers trigger a rage reaction, however, they will always be associated with primitive affect and an attack on the self. I shall consider each of these ideas in turn.

Kernberg (1992) sees rage as a primary affective state. Based on his theory of affects, rage is one of the affective states on which psychological drives are based. In other words, the libidinal and aggressive drives are organized around the individual's affective system. He also believes that even very primitive affects have a corresponding cognitive and object relational component. It is the impression that 'peak-affects' have on the infant that determine how an object is internalized.

For Kernberg, the hatred that is derived from rage is a key factor in the formation of pathological states. In his words:

> Hatred derives from rage, the primary affect around which the drive of aggression clusters; in severe psychopathology, hatred may evolve into an overwhelming dominance directed against the self as well as against others. It is a complex affect that may become the major component of the aggressive drive, overshadowing other universally present aggressive affects such as envy and disgust.
>
> (Kernberg, 1992, p.21)

Hatred is therefore only distinguishable from rage in that it is a more stable and fundamentally integrated part of the personality. Kernberg believes that rage, as a normal affective state, is transformed into hatred through traumatic attachment to a frustrating mother. Most object-relations theorists would broadly agree with this (for example Fairbairn, 1952; Guntrip, 1968; Bion, 1962b; Winnicott, 1965). They all show, in different ways, how rage need not be directly expressed and can exist in a split-off encapsulated state, greatly influencing the structure of the personality.

Kernberg understands the entrapping and consuming nature of rage as being not only due to the intensity of the affective state, but also as a consequence of the object relationship that this attachment brings. This occurs when the infant identifies both with the damaged self and the persecutory object, leaving him feeling abandoned by all good objects and trapped in a traumatizing bad-object relationship.

When one considers the phenomenology of rage, its overwhelming nature and its apparent random action, one may conclude that it is an 'objectless state'. In other words, any unsuspecting individual may suddenly become the victim of a rage attack, violent or non-violent. This, however, is not the case. Again, Kernberg (1992) is clear on this issue:

> A full-fledged rage reaction – its overwhelming nature, its diffuseness, its 'blurring' of specific cognitive contents and corresponding object relations – may convey the erroneous idea that rage is a 'pure' affect. Clinically, however, the analysis of rage reactions – as of other intense affective states – always reveals an underlying conscious or unconscious fantasy that includes a specific relation between an aspect of the self and an aspect of a significant other.
>
> (Kernberg, 1992, p.22)

Here, Kernberg draws on the Kleinian understanding of there always being an object relationship evident in all psychic states, no matter how primitive. This has important implications for understanding the type of rage that occurs in explosive acts of murder. As will be explored more thoroughly later, due to the phenomenology of rage, formulations regarding rage-type murder often make use of concepts that emphasize the cathartic nature of the act and the corresponding collapse of structural aspects of the ego. Here, the explosive release of affect is seen as a central motivating factor behind rage reactions. Too much emphasis on the discharge of affect, however, tends to distract our attention away from the kind of object relations that may contribute to such reactions. It also diverts our attention away from how the generation, or build-up of hate, occurs (Gaylin, 1984). This, in itself, appears to reflect a key function of rage. Metaphorically speaking, the overwhelming wall of affect that is expressed in a rage reaction aims to prevent any further understanding or vision of what lies behind it.

The function of rage within particular fantasies depends on the developmental level of the object. Rage at the most primitive level of object relations is used to remove immediately a source of extreme psychic pain and later, to eliminate any obstacles that stand in the way of gratification. Where the fantasies are more elaborate they include the will to reinstate all-good objects as dominant. Still later, in mature development, when the infant is able to identify with an all-good object, rage can be used as a way of asserting autonomy so as to move away from damaging bad-object relations. At this level, rage becomes far more specific in its object selection; it is more adaptive in nature and far less entrapping.

Apart from being an expression of primitive affect–object relationships, rage reactions have also been associated with elements of self-consciousness, shame and narcissistic injury. This appears to point to a particular type of self–object dynamic that leaves the self suddenly exposed, attacked and defenceless, distinguishing rage reactions from other forms of aggression.

Using a somewhat narrower definition of rage, Lewis (1993) attempts to distinguish between anger and rage reactions in his experimental observations of infants of different ages. He observes that anger is the result of the obstruction of goal-directed behaviour. Anger, according to him, emerges in relation to action aimed at overcoming barriers. It usually begins to emerge in infants of 4 months when they have discovered cause–effect relationships. Rage, on the other hand, is different because it requires *personal insult*. As this requires a degree of self-awareness, it is not present in this form until the child is 2 years of age.

One of the implications of this argument is that anger is seen to be more focused on the object, whereas rage pertains primarily to the self. Rage, Lewis argues, is 'less related to overcoming an obstacle and more related to an attack on the self as object; it is a response to an injury to the self. As such, it is more intense, less focused, and longer lasting'(p.159).

From a developmental perspective, both Lewis (1993) and Parens (1993) conclude that temper tantrums in infancy resemble a disorganized form of anger, whereas rage in children over the age of 2 and in adulthood is related to shame-filled emotions and the vulnerable exposure of the self. In Lewis' (1993) words, 'rage is a response to humiliation, a threat to the self-esteem and well-being of the individual' (p.165).

Along similar lines Retzinger (1987) writes about a cycle of rage that oscillates between rage and shame. He views anger as a simple primitive bodily response. Rage, on the other hand, appears to assume a complex psychic process where there is a focus on self-consciousness attached to an object whose presence induces shame and humiliation. Importantly the phenomenology of humiliation and shame, a sense of exposure with no support, appears to induce an isolating and entrapping sense that then erupts into rage.

There appears to be wide agreement that rage is a reaction to perceived self-damage, shame or narcissistic injury (Chessick, 1993; Kohut, 1972; Lewis, 1993; Morrison, 1989; Parens, 1993; Schafer, 1997; Shengold, 1991). Feelings of shame induce a sudden loss of self-esteem that, in turn, produces desperate defensive action aimed at preventing further humiliation. Schafer (1997) explores the underlying fantasies related to the emotional experiences of humiliation and mortification, both extreme forms of shame. He links these painful experiences to fantasies of debasement and annihilation 'associated with fantasies of deserving to die, being made to die, even causing oneself to die' (p.109). Shame is thus felt to have a deathly presence. In this context rage erupts as a defensive response to the threat of self-annihilation with the aim of destroying the perceived annihilator.

Kohut (1972) used the term 'narcissistic rage' to refer to this form of affective expression. He saw rage as a destructive form of aggression distinguishable from mature uses of aggression, which he preferred to called *self-assertive ambition*. He thought of self-assertiveness as belonging to a separate line of development originating from transformation of the *grandiose-exhibitionistic self* also responsible for the regulation of self-esteem.

Kohut maintained that all drives and motivations are firmly embedded in a self-structure. It is when the cohesiveness of this self-structure is lost that narcissistic rage arises, rendering the self most vulnerable to feelings of shame, humiliation and ridicule. For Kohut this vulnerability has a particular source leading to narcissistic injury. He explains:

> The most intense experiences of shame and the most violent forms of narcissistic rage arise in those individuals for whom a sense of absolute control over an archaic environment is indispensable because the maintenance of self-esteem – and indeed the self – depends on the unconditional availability of the approving-mirroring selfobject or of the merger-permitting idealized one.
>
> (Kohut, 1972, pp.644–5).

Thus rage emerges with sudden realizations of a lapse in the control, fantasized or real, of mirroring or idealizing objects. It is also, according to Kohut, from this kind of injury that the deepest sense of revenge, and the unrelenting aim of undoing past hurts, come. It follows then that rage reactions emerge out of a narcissistic object relationship ultimately having a self-preservative function. This is not difficult to imagine, especially if one sees narcissism, love of the self, as part of the self-preservative instincts (Glasser, 1997).

In sum, I have tried to show that rage has a number of intrapsychic correlates and is not simply an aberrant 'objectless' impulse. Rage emerges from a complex set of affect–object relationships which differ in their aim depending on the level of development. At all levels, however, rage is a response to unpleasure. It is not necessarily pathological or destructive. It is only once sustained damage to the self has occurred that rage becomes excessive and pathological, often forming a key source of self-expression. Here it has destructive intentions where an intolerable sense of shame and self-exposure are key triggers. In essence, rage is a narcissistic emotion that has self-protection at its core.

It remains to be seen how this notion of rage relates to the act of rage-type murder. I hope to show that there are a number of intrapsychic factors that force part of the psyche into an encapsulated state where – although leaving one with a picture of 'normality' and even non-aggressiveness – it is at its most lethal. It is this part of the psyche that, if exposed, unleashes an annihilatory sense of shame that has devastating consequences. I now turn to consider some of the defining features of violence.

VIOLENCE

Violence, as opposed to aggression, has received relatively little attention in psychoanalysis. Usually, when it is considered, it is only considered in the therapeutic context where fantasies of violence rather than actual acts of violence are explored. As mentioned earlier, only recently, with contributions from Fonagy and Target (1995), Glasser (1998), Hyatt-Williams (1998), Meloy (1992), Gilligan

(1996) and Perelberg (1999a), have intrapsychic factors associated with violent behaviour been more thoroughly explored.

Glasser (1998) restricts his definition of violence to 'a bodily response with an intended infliction of bodily harm on another person' (p.887). The focus here is on the breach of the bodily boundary. Violence towards inanimate figures, as well as unconscious forms of violence, he argues, have different psychodynamic pathways and symbolic meanings. Shengold (1999) views violence more generally as the loss of control of the aggressive impulses leading to action. Others, such as Mitchell (1993), Meers (1982) and Buie et al. (1983), have chosen to emphasize the psychic motivation behind the act as key to defining violent behaviour, rather than the physical bodily encounter itself. Limentani (1991) appears to take the middle ground between these two, claiming that an act is only violent if the individual shows a clear intention to do physical damage to an object.

Clearly there are many different ways in which one could define what constitutes an act of violence. This has led to some authors distinguishing between different kinds of violence. Lefer (1984), for instance, describes four different types of violence: violence used as a means to an end with no need for justification; violence that is a means to an end but is justified; violence that occurs because of a dissociated state; and violence that, through a position of power, emanates from a symbiotic relationship with either the first or second type of violence-prone individual. The last type is most interesting in that Lefer acknowledges that situational factors may play an important role in some forms of violent behaviour. I see this as a defining dimension of all forms of violence, with the nature of the situation, its effects and impact, varying across different violent behaviours. We shall return to this in the next chapter.

For my purpose, I will define the *act* of violence as the physical show, or actualization, of aggression, leading to the destruction or damage of an object. This view is similar to Meloy's (1988) definition that violence includes anything that involves 'the inflicting of physical damage on persons or property' (p.388). It is the physical and destructive nature of the act that separates it from other intrapsychic or interpersonal activity.

In keeping with the general idea that aggression may have different sources and psychodynamic pathways, general distinctions between types of violence have been suggested based on a similar argument. In broad terms, although opinions differ about underlying dynamics, a distinction is usually made between what might be called *object-centred violence* and *self-centred violence*. In the former, violence is primarily aimed at destruction or damage of the object. The latter refers to violence that is, at its core, self-protective. Perhaps the most recent and significant distinctions made along these lines have been put forward by Mervin Glasser and Reid Meloy.

Glasser (1998) distinguishes between *self-preservative* and *sado-masochistic violence*, bearing some resemblance to Fromm's (1973) earlier distinction between *defensive* and *destructive aggression*. Glasser describes self-preservative violence as the psychological derivative of the 'fight or flight' response that occurs in the presence of danger. He views this as being close to what can be regarded as an automatic instinctual response and thus it differs from Freud's (1920) idea of a separate death instinct. He makes use of Freud's (1915) initial conceptualization of aggression here, where aggression emerges as an ego-instinct. Although the ego perceives the threat, it is a far more primitive reactive impulse that actually attacks. This form of violence usually occurs in reaction to a perceived attack on the self or a narcissistic injury. According to Glasser (1998), it 'focuses on the dangerousness of the object, rather than the object itself' (p.888). Thus the response of the object is of little interest and the aim of the violence is to eliminate perceived danger. For Glasser, aggression is a psychic response existing along a continuum with self-preservative violence at its extreme. On the other end of the continuum the 'aggressive response is carried out psychically' (p.890), whether the threat is real or imagined, and bodily expression is no longer required to eliminate danger.

Sado-masochistic violence, on the other hand, has its origins in the libidiniza-tion of self-preservative violence. The perpetrator obtains pleasure from violence inflicted and thus the fate of the object – that the object suffers – becomes impor-tant in this form of violence. He argues that libidinization, by definition, converts self-preservative violence into sadistic violence, making fantasy and object relations key ingredients in this form of violence. The aim here is to preserve the object and to make it suffer. Further, in contrast to self-preservative violence, anxiety is usually absent.

Meloy (1992) draws a distinction between *predatory violence* and *affective violence*. He also puts forward two other dimensions that cut across these types of violence. The first dimension is the level of reality testing that the individual is capable of before, or during, the violence. The second refers to the nature of 'object selection' that occurs in the violent individual. He bases his distinction not only on psychodynamic and behavioural factors, but also on neuropsychological evidence that suggests that different neuro-anatomical pathways are used in the two different types of violence.

Affective violence emerges in response to an internal or external threat where-by the autonomic nervous system is activated leading to a defensive response. This is similar to Glasser's self-preservative violence; both appear to describe the rage-type reaction that leads to violence. They disagree, however, when it comes to their second categorizations of violence (Glasser, 1999; Meloy, 1999).

According to Meloy, predatory aggression refers, in its extreme form, to psychopathic forms of violence where a clear motive, planning, and a degree of emotional detachment before, and during, the act are evident. In his words, a 'suspension of empathic regard' (p.390) takes place. This differs from what Glasser identifies as sado-masochistic violence in that predatory violence need not necessarily be sadistic. 'Predatory' is also perhaps an unfortunate word to use for this class of violence because the word, as Glasser (1998) points out, is associ-ated more with animal predation where the function of violence – to survive – is essentially self-preservative. Meloy and Glasser also disagree on how their categorizations of violence are related. Whilst Glasser argues that sado-masochistic violence emerges out of what are initially self-preservative acts, Meloy sees them as distinctly different. He accuses Glasser of ignoring empirical research in this area and argues that self-preservative and sado-masochistic violence undergo different psychobiological paths of development and are in no way linked (Meloy, 1999).

It is difficult to argue that either of these approaches is more accurate, as they arise from very different perspectives on the topic. There is little doubt that the above categories define particular types of violence. These categories, however, should not be seen as discrete. Not all psychopathic forms of violence are sadistic for instance, and not all rage attacks lack sadistic or predatory tendencies. Glasser's typology allows for some flexibility here as sadistic violence and self-preservative violence are seen as linked. Meloy's theory, however, is not in keeping with these observations.

These categories also do not appear adequately to explain all forms of violence. For instance, how should we understand ritual violence, suicide, or socially accepted forms of violence. It appears that in these situations other factors take precedence over the typologies being put forward here.

A number of different psychodynamic factors underlie the violent act, each in some way explaining why aggression turns into violence. Gilligan (1996), for instance, in his work with high-security inmates, convincingly shows how a deep sense of shame is central to understanding the flight into violence. Gilligan, in fact, is convinced that all forms of violence have shame at their core. Perelberg (1995a), on the other hand, focuses on a core phantasy associated with the primal scene as being a primary precondition for violence. Clearly different authors have concentrated on different factors that might lead to violence. Intrapsychic conditions would also be different depending on the type of violent act committed. For this reason, I think a dimensional approach to understanding the role of intrapsychic factors and their link to violence is useful.

Implicit in many accounts of violence is the assumption that high levels of aggression are closer to the eruption of physical violence. However, no such linear relationship between aggression and violence appears to exist. The show of violence is mediated by a number of intrapsychic factors such as the type of defences used, the nature of phantasy and capacity for mentalization or representation. In short, whether aggression turns into violence is best understood as being dependent on the configuration of a number of these factors that I shall now explore in detail.

Chapter 2

Seven intrapsychic dimensions of violence

Working with violent individuals in both therapeutic and research settings, I have found it useful to conceptualize different forms of violence as having distinguishing intrapsychic features that can be viewed along a number of intrapsychic dimensions. Such dimensions coincide in a particular way, at a specific point in time, to determine the kind of violence expressed. Aside from being a means of classifying violent behaviour through exploring these intrapsychic factors, certain dimensions also appear to be more prominent than others, depending on the type of violence discussed. For instance, poor representational capacity appears to be a prominent feature of explosive violence, but does little to explain why sadistic violence occurs.

Each of the following dimensions holds within it a partial theory of violence. In doing so, the dimensional approach moves towards offering various explanations as to why violence occurs, and further, why it may occur in some situations and not in others. The main question here is how, and why, does aggression in some cases turn into violence? Lefer (1984) calls this 'the fine edge of violence' and asks; 'Why can one individual be incipiently violent [aggressive in my terms] but stop short of physically hurting another person and another feel no restraints against injuring people physically?'(p.253). Each dimension offers only a partial answer to this question.

I shall consider seven different, but inter-related, dimensions underlying the violent act. In reviewing some of the main contributions in this area, I confine myself to those analytic authors who have written particularly about actual physical violence and draw less on those who are writing solely about a psychological construct. The intrapsychic dimensions to be discussed here are: the nature and quality of object relationships; representational capacity; brutalization of the self; sexuality; the role of phantasy/fantasy; defensive organizations; and interaction with the external situation.

It is not my intention here to put forward comprehensive explanations as to how these dimensions apply to different categories of violence. My main purpose is to set out the seven dimensions and outline the central dilemmas and scope of each one in order to lay the groundwork for the analysis of rage-type murder. I shall only draw on other forms of violence to illustrate the range of the different dimensions discussed. It should also be said that the dearth of psychodynamic research in this area leaves many gaps in our knowledge as far as specific acts of violence are concerned and how they feature within these dimensions.

SEVEN INTRAPSYCHIC DIMENSIONS

The nature and quality of the object world

It is often held that violence occurs when aggressive or sadistic object relations are simply enacted towards the outside world. Here, there is some consistency between the person that is targeted and the individual's object relations. This, however, is not always the case, especially in defensive, explosive, or group-sanctioned forms of violence. The role of the object relations and the target of violence in these cases is far more difficult to fathom.

Meloy (1988) raises important questions here about the nature and quality of the object/s associated with the intrapsychic make-up of the violent individual. Notably, he wonders about the role of affect in understanding 'violent' object relations and whether we should distinguish between objectless and object-related violence? Secondly, are there particular internal objects/part-objects that instigate a violent outcome? Thirdly, how defined and complex are these internalizations, and how are they related to the individual's object world and the self? There are a number of consistent findings related to these questions.

Capacity for object relating

The capacity for object relating in potentially violent individuals is often observed as being ostensibly unproblematic (Hering, 1997; Hyatt-Williams, 1998). This may be because primitive object relations are often hidden behind more mature defences such as repression. This might also be understood in terms of a battle between more realistically oriented parts of the psyche and destructive 'objectless' states. Hering (1997), for instance, argues that acts of violence occur when destructive parts of the personality hijack object-seeking parts that had previously developed the capacity to distinguish between good and bad:

> These faculties of the mature and sane part of the personality, along with these best capacities for realistic and responsible thinking, are sucked into the maelstrom of a relentless 'evil' propaganda and are enlisted to loyally serve a fanatical pursuit of destruction while, at the same time, maintaining the resemblance of a benign ordinary life.
>
> (Hering, 1997, p.212)

This kind of formulation has been observed in a number of studies, most using

Winnicott's idea of the False Self which we shall return to later (Gallwey, 1985; Glasser, 1998). Does this mean, however, that some violent behaviour is essentially 'objectless'? Although some have argued that emotionally charged rage reactions are 'objectless' in nature, as argued earlier in discussing rage, this is a deceptive assumption. We observed that it is reasonably well established that this form of violence is aimed at the elimination of the object, where the fate of the object *per se* is unimportant. This in itself may lead to the faulty assumption that internal objects are less important in this form of violence. Further, the act itself, often being a poorly focused explosive outburst, does appear at first glance to be 'objectless'. The individual's inability to explain his own rage, which is often the case, may also lead one in this direction.

Given, however, that a majority of violent individuals do not suffer from chronic psychotic disorders, their capacity for object relating and the ability to differentiate between objects is often relatively intact. In these cases, it appears more accurate to say that this state is induced by a high degree of unarticulated affect that overwhelms the object world (Meloy, 1988). Further support for this can be taken from the fact that these acts are very seldom randomly targeted acts. There still remains, prior to the act, a pattern of object selection that can be traced to internal factors. It is only in rare cases, when such affective forms of violence are random and completely unprovoked (Sohn, 1995), that a more chronic lack of object relatedness can be assumed. Even here, it is not that object relating is completely absent, it is more that object representations are poorly defined.

What of the capacity for object relating in sadistic forms of violence? A particular form of perverted relationship with the object is needed to perpetuate sadistic violence. There appears to be relative agreement that dehumanization of the object is a key factor here. To be sure, some have argued that a process of dehumanization of the object world needs to take place if any type of violence is to occur (Kutash, 1978; Lefer, 1984). Perelberg (1995b) has further argued that dehumanization can also be used as a defence to protect the individual from the frustrations and violence of the human world. It essentially implies an expected lack of empathy for objects and is most characteristically observed in antisocial personalities.

Dehumanization, however, is used differently to refer to the internal world of the sadistic psychopath. In these cases there is a preoccupation with the survival, death and resurrection of the object. It does not mean that the object's response to feeling is not an important factor, as might automatically be assumed. Making the object suffer and feel pain is a primary dynamic behind the violence. It is felt to be exciting and stimulating to the perpetrator. Lefer (1984) explains this as a process that arises out of a deadened sense of self: 'The violent one may have completely deadened feelings, feel depersonalized, and envy the capacity of others to feel. Only when violent may he feel pleasure and stimulation' (p.256). He goes on to say that violence occurs here because the individual hungers for a human bond that is affected by violent interaction through which he acquires a kind of recognition of his impact on the individual.

Biven (1997) is in agreement with this line of thinking. He reserves the term *dehumanizing principle* for 'a small group of individuals that has been irrevocably traumatized' (p.24) and display sadistic violent tendencies. Arguing from a more traditional Freudian standpoint, Biven (1997) claims that this occurs when trauma disrupts the developmental task of gaining a sense of mastery over the object world. It blocks a healthy expression of aggression which is diverted from the world of human contact, taking refuge in an inanimate object world where the individual seeks stimulation rather than comfort.

Before considering how particular internal object relations impact on violent propensities, the distinction often made between preoedipal and oedipal psychic processes requires brief elucidation. Often the term 'preoedipal' is used to refer to a more primitive stage of development leading to assumptions that different pathological states are either preoedipal *or* oedipal in nature because they all lie on a developmental continuum. This also informs the misconception that preoedipal experience always leads to more extreme manifestations of pathology (Westen, 1989). In my view, however, these modes of experience do not exist along a simple developmental continuum as the term 'preoedipal' suggests. My views are similar to those of Grotstein (1981) and Ogden (1992) in so far as they see oedipal and preoedipal modes of generating experience as operating in a synchronic fashion. Although there is a developmental link between preoedipal and oedipal processes in that one dominates the other depending on the stage of development, they essentially belong to different modes, or tracks, of experience. Here, oedipal experience, triadic object relations, conflict, object-oriented experience and other associated features exist alongside preoedipal experience generated by dyadic object relations and issues related to narcissism and deficits in the self.

Viewed in this way, the external world is experienced on two different registers. It is more accurate, in this sense, to view pathological states as being a consequence of vulnerability experienced in one of the two areas, or as a result of a breakdown in the dialectic between the two. In other words, vulnerability in one area does not exclude other modes of experience, even though this will obviously impact on other parts of the psyche. Borderline patients, for instance, are often thought to be dominated by preoedipal concerns, but this should not be taken to mean that they are incapable of oedipal experience; both modes of experience are always apparent to some extent.

This model has many conceptual implications. For instance, the often debated separation of conflict-based and deficit-based pathological states no longer applies here as conflict and deficit are seen as inseparable. In essence, the one causes the other. I do not wish to expand on these ideas here. I merely intend to introduce this way of thinking to sketch a context for understanding oedipal and preoedipal concerns related to the propensity to commit violent acts. Violence is not generated solely out of oedipal or preoedipal intrapsychic precipitants. In keeping with the previous chapter about 'many aggressions', vulnerabilities or impairments in both may induce violence when the situation is right. It also does not necessarily follow that preoedipal vulnerabilities would lead to more extreme forms of violence. We shall return to this reasoning in exploring sexuality as a dimension of violence. For the time being I simply wish to point out that in making reference to preoedipal concerns in future discussions I do not mean to imply that such individuals do not struggle with oedipal conflicts as well. Second, in keeping with the above conceptualization, my use of the terms 'primitive' and 'preoedipal' does not delineate a discrete developmental stage but rather describes a mode of experience. Rather than simply referring to a developmental level, the word 'primitive' means a system of narcissistic object relations where the distinction between self and other are not clearly defined.

So far we have discussed some of the dynamic processes found to be apparent in the object world of the violent individual. I turn now to considering a number of important contributions towards understanding the role of key internalized objects in violent individuals.

The primary maternal object

Perelberg (1999a), in her introduction to a number of psychoanalytic case studies on violence and suicide, points out that a central organizing dynamic that precipitates violence occurs when the self is overwhelmed or consumed by an object. Meloy (1992) adds to this the idea that, for the perpetrator, the object possesses some internalized sense of identity. He refers to this when he writes about the fear of being trapped 'in an identity-bearing introject' (p.8). Here, the violent response essentially functions as a desperate means of creating space between self and the object. Although this is the aim, it is complicated by the fact that the primary identification that has occurred makes the maternal presence inescapably a part of the self and thus cannot simply be rejected. Many have located the origins of this dynamic between infant and mother where a pathological attachment, symbiosis or fusion, causes complications in the child's sense of identity and separateness (Duncan and Duncan, 1978; Glasser, 1998; Hyatt-Williams, 1998; Kernberg, 1984; Shengold, 1989).

The role of the overprotective mother often emerges in the literature (Bateman, 1999; Perelberg, 1995b; Shengold, 1993). Glasser (1998) refers to a situation of over-gratification leading to an absence of a clearly defined dyadic object relationship. In an earlier paper (Glasser, 1997), he explains how narcissistic relating between mother and infant leads to a basic core complex: a dilemma between feeling consumed or abandoned by the mother. This leads to a split in the maternal object, the avaricious and the rejecting mother, which, in turn, cause fears of annihilation. Feeling either engulfed or rejected by the mother, the infant has two defensive options: retreat into a narcissistic state or use self-preservative aggression against the obliterating mother. Using his distinction between two types of violence, mentioned earlier, Glasser separates this form of violence from sadistic types where oedipal dynamics are more evident.

Shengold (1991) writes about a similar type of narcissistic object relationship that contains violent propensities. He finds that maternal over-stimulation, combined with the child being treated as an extension of the mother, leads to what he calls *soul murder*. Here, the infant's self is smothered and replaced by the mother's idealizations. Once these inevitably falter, the child is left exposed to the dread of having nothing after being promised an ideal world. This in turn leads to a devastating sense of having no self. Lefer (1984) identifies a similar dynamic in the transferences of individuals who had committed murder. He observed that such offenders would most typically display idealized parental transferences. Any slight indication of perceived abandonment, however, evoked extremely negative transferences which he associates with potential violence.

From an attachment theory perspective, following Bowlby (1969), some have emphasized the importance of primary attachments in exploring violent behaviour. Meloy (1992) points out that most acts of violence take place within an existing attachment. This is one of his motivations for using attachment theory to understand different forms of violence. He argues that disorders of extreme detachment, when no stable attachment occurs, are the bedrock of the psychopathic personality where a chronic lack of emotion towards human objects is apparent and no clear internalization of a maternal object occurs. The mother is felt to have abandoned the child and is lost to him, eventually leading to a sense of detachment with little protest.

Zulueta (1993) emphasizes the role of trauma and deprivation as being the most prominent factor in abnormal attachments that lead to violence. Apart from having to deal with the loss of the object's love, however, a less emphasized problem here is the loss of the object's assistance in countering unknown inner forces (Hitchcock, 1996). In agreement with an emphasis on object loss, some have argued that many of the most heinous acts of murder involving mutilation and intended suffering appear to be primitive re-enacted attempts at dealing with the loss of a primary object (Biven, 1997; Harris and Pontius, 1975; Hyatt-Williams, 1998; Zulueta, 1993).

At the other end of the spectrum, disorders of extreme attachment form one of the main predisposing factors for other forms of violence. However, problems of attachment here are less obvious because they are often perceived as normal in society and thus go undetected (Meloy, 1992). Most of the psychodynamic characteristics emerge from the *rapprochement* sub-phase of Mahler's separation-individuation phase of development. This occurs at approximately the age of 18 months where a growing uneasiness about being away from the mother is felt. It becomes difficult to relinquish infantile omnipotence giving rise to separation anxiety, feelings of shame and abandonment rage akin to anxieties most evident in the borderline personality structure.

In keeping with the idea that the mode of attachment influences violent behaviour, Shoham *et al.* (1997) found, in a study using a prison sample, that attachment to family was associated with the type of violence committed. They argue that those more attached to family were more likely to commit impulsive acts of violence whilst those who did not receive any form of punishment during childhood were more likely to commit planned acts of violence.

In sum, although seen in different ways, all the above note problems with separation from the maternal object as being a key correlate in violent individuals. Further, there appears to be wide agreement that defensive violence occurs from within an extreme attachment dynamic. I shall explore this further in relation to my work with rage-type murderers.

The paternal or third object

Viewing the paternal object as the third object, bringing with it internal space and the capacity to symbolize, is not a new formulation specific to understanding violent individuals. This understanding essentially begins with Freud's (1923) notion of the superego and has been developed considerably by a number of psychoanalysts. A fair amount has been written about the role and internalization of the father in potentially violent individuals (Bateman, 1999; Britton, 1992; Fonagy and Target, 1995; Gaddini, 1992; Limentani, 1991; Perelberg, 1999a; Stoller, 1979). In most cases the paternal object is found to be an intermediary object breaking a pathological symbiosis or fusion between self and the primary object. The paternal object is felt to be less of a threat as it is less contaminated by projections of hate and envy. Therefore it follows that the absence of a coherent paternal introject is often isolated as one of the key problems with violent individuals. Perelberg (1999a), in her review of a number of studies of potentially violent individuals, finds this to be a common occurrence. In her words: 'Each patient felt trapped in a dyadic relationship with the mother/analyst where the perspective of the father as a third object was lacking' (p.8).

Campbell (1999), referring particularly to the pre-suicide state as violence turned against the body, views the father's role as enabling the child to dis-identify from the mother. This, in turn, allows the child to occupy a place in the father's mind separate from the mother. He follows this dynamic in an interesting case study where he is able to identify, through enactment, his own failure to rescue his patient from a murderous mother imago. His failure leads to a plea for a third object, the father-therapist in this case, to stand in the way of regression to a more violent and entrapping sado-masochistic transference.

Aggression and envy towards the paternal object may also precipitate violence. Fonagy and Target (1995) argue that destroying the tie between the parental couple as part of an oedipal dynamic is not always the key motivation behind violence. The father is important in that he represents the possibility of reflection. Attacks on the paternal object thus involve destroying his awareness of the infantile self that has essentially been ignored by the mother. Contrary to an oedipal understanding, this kind of violence against the paternal object is more concerned with destroying a witness than destroying a rival.

Does this mean that more primitive internalizations of the father are more apparent in violent individuals? This may be the case in some forms of violence. For instance, Abrahamsen (1973) and Perelberg (1999b) have noted the precarious nature of male identifications or internal representations. In a number of cases

Perelberg observes that there are often rapid oscillations between male and female identifications in violent individuals, making it difficult for them to establish a cohesive identity. She isolates identification with the female object and its association with passivity as a trigger that could evoke terror and possible violence in her male patients. This appears to be a prominent feature in chronic domestic offenders where a fragile male identity is maintained through repetitive violence and control in order to deflect having to identify with a female object. In working with abusers of this kind, it becomes apparent that they find themselves trapped in a double bind situation: they either identify with the aggressor, causing considerable shame and self-hate, or they face chronic insecurity and threat because they have an impaired capacity to identify with other male figures that is due to the terror they themselves have suffered in the past. Either way, their identifications remain unstable, making 'female' identifications a greater threat. In the later case, I have found that these kinds of precarious identification with male objects are more akin to 'imitation' (Gaddini, 1992), than to identification proper. This is part of a more primitive process involving the imitation of the object rather than its internalization, which makes the individual far more dependent on the object always being present. In individuals who are particularly fragile, violence may often occur when separation puts the object out of reach and, as a consequence, the imitation process fails.

Although these preoedipal processes are of utmost importance in understanding violence, violence may also emerge from oedipal themes such as jealousy, rivalry and revenge. The extent to which these themes would be translated into violent action, however, appears to be more dependent on the other dimensions of violence to be explored here. For instance, whether an individual becomes violent because of some rivalrous act, like competing for a lover, would depend on situational factors at the time, his capacity to think through his actions, or whether the individual had a past history of being victimized.

Continuing with elements of 'thirdness' in the psyche, what can be said of the role of the superego in violent offenders? The traditional superego results from identification with the same-sex parent in order to avert castration anxiety in the boy and loss of love in the girl (Freud, 1923). It has been understood in many different ways since then (Chasseguet-Smirgel, 1984; Fenichel, 1945; Glasser, 1978; Klein, 1927; Lacan, 1977; O'Shaughnessy, 1999; Rosenfeld, 1952; Steiner, 1993). I will not discuss these specific details here. Broadly, the superego represents the internalization of parental values, goals and restrictions. It represents the conscience of the individual that could be either punitive, absent or supportive. The status of the superego in violent individuals appears to vary. As previously discussed, the superego is often seen as absent in psychopathic or criminal forms of violence, but is overly restrictive and harsh in explosive violence.

Freud (1923) believed the superego to be absent in psychopaths. Fenichel (1931), however, argued that although extreme psychopaths have not developed a superego, most do have some primitive superego capacity, but it is ineffective. The argument for the underdevelopment of the superego in delinquents and psychopaths has received considerable support. Many of these individuals come from loveless families where there is a frequent absence of the father and hence the capacity to develop an adequate superego is compromised.

Klein (1927), on the other hand, saw the superego as being extremely harsh and punitive in cases of violence. This was consistent with her ideas about the archaic formation of the superego. From this point of view violence is understood as a form of externalization. It is a means of alleviating an inner persecution that occurs between the ego and punitive superego. Violence serves to reassure the ego that harsh inner attacks can be outdone by controlling and attacking the external world. Klein understood this to work alongside an unconscious sense of guilt caused by the superego. The latter is similar to Freud's (1916) understanding of criminal behavior as being the enactment of unconscious guilt. Symington (1996) finds this to be important, specifically in violent situations, as opposed to general criminal conduct. Violence erupts, he argues, when unconscious guilt, as a result of internal attacks on the ego, becomes intolerable.

Much could be said about how different analysts conceptualize the superego. Further exploration of how these conceptualizations relate to physical acts of violence is still required. For instance, I have found Glasser's (1978) distinction between the *proscribed* and *prescribed* superego to be useful in its application to different forms of violence. The later represents the goals and ideals of the individual, whereas the former approximates his or her conscience or morals. It might be argued that some forms of violence are more closely associated with proscribed aspects of the superego, whereas others may best be related to prescribed qualities. In socially sanctioned acts of violence, for example, one would expect to find inflated aspects of the proscribed superego to be partially responsible for initiating 'justified' violence. In such cases the prescribed superego may be variable or have no influence at all on the violent outcome. On the other hand, psychopathic forms of violence rely on diminished capacities in both sections of the superego where prescribed aspects are often perverted so that 'negative' goals and actions are viewed as rewarding. We shall return to this distinction in exploring my understanding of the rage-type offender.

Representational capacity

Representational capacity evolves from the transformation of somatic excitation into psychically derived drives, objects and affects. Lecours and Bouchard (1997) describe this process as follows:

> The process of mentalization refers to a preconscious/ego linking function, consisting of a connecting of bodily excitations with endopsychic representations. In one sense, mentalization could be seen as the necessary mediator between the ego and the id, yet in another, it serves as a necessary *creation* of a psychic id.

(Lecours and Bouchard, 1997, pp.855–6)

A number of psychoanalysts argue that the capacity for violence is related to an inability to mentalize (Bion, 1962a; Fonagy *et al.*, 1993a; Fonagy and Target, 1995; Hyatt-Williams, 1996, 1998; Segal, 1997). In essence, they argue that the inability to form coherent internal object representations causes a confusion between body and mind, the mental and the physical. Implicit in this is the idea that physical acts provide a more immediate outlet for drive–affect expression, an idea well established by Freud himself. In 'Inhibitions, symptoms and anxiety' (Freud, 1926), for instance, he states: 'Touching and physical contact are the immediate aim of the aggressive as well as the loving object cathexes' (p.122). Earlier, in 'Formulations on the two principles of mental functioning' (Freud, 1911), he explains how, through a process of binding (*bundig*), free-floating excitations are transformed into psychological elements mediating the concrete immediate needs of instinctual life.

The implications of this line of thinking have perhaps been most thoroughly explored by Wilfred Bion (1958, 1962a, 1962b, 1963, 1970). His understanding of the nature of β-elements and the α-function, as well as the container–contained relationship, among other concepts, has contributed greatly to understanding the process of thinking and thought formation. An important implication of this theoretical standpoint is that the unconscious is no longer viewed as pre-formed and symbolic. Some degree of psychic elaboration needs to occur before repression, as it is traditionally understood, can operate. These ideas have laid the foundation for a number of recent contributions to understanding the impact of the representational system on violence. Fonagy and his colleagues have developed this line of thinking considerably and I turn now to consider some of their findings.

Fonagy *et al.* (1993a) draw a distinction between the *pre-reflective self* and the *reflective self*. The former is synonymous with the experiencing physical body, whereas the latter is the 'internal observer of mental life' (p.472). In their view, reflective capacity is acquired through interaction:

> The child's growing recognition of the importance of mental states (feeling, beliefs, desires and intentions) arises through the shared understanding of his own mental world and that of his caregiver. She reflects upon the infant's mental experience and re-presents it to him ... Her role is to provide a creative social mirror which can capture for the infant aspects of his activity and then add an organizing perspective.
>
> (Fonagy *et al.*, 1993a, p.473)

Fonagy and his colleagues liken this to Winnicott's idea of *cross-identifications* where the infant's mental space is acquired through careful observation of his own mental life and a primary identification with the caregiver's reflective capacity. His own acquired reflective capabilities provide the individual with a sense of himself as a mental entity.

Violence, they believe, originates from an inability to reflect or understand the mental state of the self and others. Here, the difference between the mental and physical diminishes:

> In the absence of adequate reflective capacity, the pre-reflective and physical self may come to substitute for mental functions – the body may reflect experiences instead of the mind and thus be imbued with thought and feeling.
>
> (Fonagy *et al.*, 1993a, p.481)

The tendency to represent mental states unconsciously in bodily terms also leads to the mind being perceived as accessible via the body (self or other). Moreover, this also reduces the individual's capacity for the inhibition of aggression as the capacity to experience real suffering in the self or in others cannot be sufficiently represented or mentalized.

Fonagy *et al.* (1991) conducted extensive research on mother–infant interactions in the first year of life. They found that parents who had difficulty reflecting on their own intentions during the research interviews were more likely to have 1-year-olds who displayed avoidance and aggression when they had to be separated from their parents. They contend that these kinds of aggressive displays are not initially pathological. They serve an adaptive function aimed at defending the psychological self from thoughts that it does not have the representational or mental capacity to protect itself from.

When the parent's reflective capacity is compromised drastically, however, the child may develop pathological forms of destructiveness. Here, aggression as a defence fails at protecting the psychological self. Aggression intensifies eventually causing a pathological fusion with the self. As a result, 'aggression becomes inextricably linked to self-expression' (Fonagy *et al.*, 1993a, p.475). This complication causes, among other solutions, the introjection of a distorted, or even absent, picture of the child as part of the mother's internal world and becomes the 'germ of a potentially persecutory object which is lodged in the self, but is alien and unassailable' (Fonagy *et al.*, 1993a, p.494).

If the capacity to conceive thoughts is poorly developed it may be used as a defence against psychic pain. Here, aggression is used as a means of turning against thoughts, representations and psychic processes that are felt to be intolerable. Fonagy *et al.* (1993a) indicate that this constitutes a 'more profound disturbance than simply the internalization of rejecting, unempathic parents' (p.481). It is not simply the internalization of an aggressive, violent or rejecting object that explains violence, it is more profoundly the representational system, the inability to mentalize, that translates into a violent solution. In support of this, in a later study, Fonagy and Target (1995) report on their involvement with a number of patients who do not fit the 'cycle of abuse profile' but display a similar fragility in their ability to mentalize. They argue that these problems arise from more subtle forms of interaction that are not easily observable in relationships with others but still threaten the psychological self.

The ability to *re*-present is also associated with the capacity for symbolic thought: the ability to allow one representation to stand for another. Violent murderous images, for instance, may stand for angry feelings towards someone and not for murder in itself. Without the capacity to re-present, however, these murderous images can only be seen and felt as concrete images, bringing them closer to being a reality. The absence of the symbolic function in violent individuals has been discussed by a number of authors (Bucci, 1998; Fonagy and Target, 1995; Hyatt-Williams, 1998; Lecours and Bouchard, 1997; Segal, 1997; Sohn, 1995). Consistent with this, Lefer (1984) observes how dream elements are often felt to be like concrete dangerous objects in the minds of violent patients, leaving them disturbed and paranoid in waking life. Dreams become what he calls fixed 'candid camera' type dreams. They themselves become concrete encapsulating objects that are felt to 'attack' the individual.

What remains important to understand is how this situation comes about and its relation to different forms of violence. In some cases this may be a chronic situation. In other healthier individuals there may be a sudden collapse in the symbolic function caused by a traumatic event. Still further, it may occur because of the destruction of the symbolic function by a sinister part of the psyche. All these possibilities exist.

Lecours and Bouchard (1997) develop a model that attempts, amongst a number of other things, to explore different levels of mental elaboration and how they may be related to violence. The degree of elaboration is dependent on the extent to which the containment of affect has occurred. At the most primitive level, what they call *disruptive impulsion*, no mental elaboration occurs. Drive–affect is expressed in an uncontrolled way and has not undergone repression because it has not been 'mentalized'. It is expressed somatically or through motor activity and gives rise to extreme forms of destructive uncontrollable violence that are crude and unfocused.

At the next level, *modulated impulsion*, there is some containment, but unarticulated affect is still evacuated from the psyche. No reflection takes place, but it serves as a cathartic release. At a more sophisticated level of mental elaboration, evacuation via the 'action defenses' (p.863) does not occur and unwanted representations or affects now undergo a process of externalization. Through externalization the individual can talk about the affective state; it is represented in some way. It is disowned through the representational system using more mature defences as opposed to 'action defences'. They do not give an indication of whether this would mean that violence, as a bodily expression, would ever occur at this level of representation.

Although the degree of mentalization appears related to the propensity for violence, it is unlikely that the entire personality will be uniformly plagued with the same problem. Perhaps, along lines similar to Bion's (1957) ideas on psychotic and non-psychotic aspects of the personality, it is more productive to think of specific parts of the personality as remaining unrepresented and unsymbolized for different reasons. For instance, in violence that has its roots in some traumatic happening, the representational system is suddenly overwhelmed by particular indigestible circumstances that cause the representational system to implode. On the other hand, focused, more intentional acts of violence may stem from a particular object relation that has remained unarticulated and closer to physical forms of expression whilst the rest of the personality makes use of the symbolic function.

Importantly, however, the collapse or incapacity of the representational system cannot explain all forms of violence. Violence that is premeditated and carefully planned or sanctioned may be construed in elaborate mentalizations that may become obsessional. Further, a central feature of sadistic violence involves an elaborate use of representational space where the capacity to imagine the victim's pain is an essential feature. In this case the representational system is inverted. Instead of moving away from bodily forms of representation, psychic images are tinged with excitement giving rise to more elaborate images. Although these kinds of mentalization may be elaborate and detailed, they usually hold very little meaning for the individual apart from their primitive excitement value. In this sense it is a *pseudo-representational system*. The excitement that such images induce is usually what drives these individuals into violent action. Once asked to explain their actions, however, they are often unable to, illustrating how devoid of real meaning these representations of self and other are. In these forms of violence it seems to me that representational capacity is less a determinant of violence and more a vehicle through which other dimensions of experience can manifest, such as brutalization of the self and the sexualization of activity. Similarly, in socially sanctioned or group violence, representational capacity plays less of a role. Apart from the complexity that group dynamics introduce in these situations, violence here is usually carried out as a form of rationalization in defence of, or as a challenge toward, some symbol of oedipal authority.

Brutalization of the self: trauma and loss

Physical or sexual abuse and other kinds of trauma are often reported in the case histories of violent individuals (Biven, 1997; Bowlby, 1969; Gilligan, 1996; Hyatt-Williams, 1996, 1998; Lefer, 1984; Zulueta, 1993). The trauma may have occurred in childhood, or result from a more contemporary event in adulthood as is the case with individuals who have suffered post-traumatic stress disorder. Further, both acute traumatic experience and what Khan (1974) called 'cumulative trauma' may render the individual more vulnerable to committing acts of violence. Often termed 'the cycle of violence', violence from this perspective is understood to emerge through a defensive identification with the aggressor, a concept first used by Anna Freud (1936). The individual identifies with the aggressor in order to escape a vulnerable abused self that is then projected into someone else. It would appear that the nature of the violence that occurs here would depend on two factors. First, as it occurs through identification, it would depend on the kind of violence to which the individual was victim. Second, it would depend on the extent to which the identification predominates in the personality. If for instance, as with Rosenfeld's (1971) description of an internal 'mafia gang', the aggressive identification becomes a structuralized part of the self, then the violence moves from being originally defensive to being a perverse means of reaffirming identity.

For Kernberg (1992), an early traumatic relationship with the mother leaves an experience of the mother as being an all-bad object that has destroyed or consumed the all-good one. In this case, destructive attempts are aimed at trying to restore good object relations. Commenting on a similar process to 'identification with the aggressor', Kernberg argues that although this leads to an imagined triumph over the sadistic traumatizing object, it also leads to a futile and entrapping intrapsychic situation. This occurs because the individual identifies with both the damaged self and the persecutory object and, as a result, is consumed by an object relationship based on hatred and aggression.

Hyatt-Williams (1998) emphasizes the role of traumatic experience in perpetuating violence from a different perspective. Using Bion's understanding of undigested mental states, he argues that traumatic experience or the loss of an object stands in the way of normal psychic digestion. Psychic states induced by trauma often cannot be contained and worked through adequately and thus cannot be mourned. As a consequence, these experiences remain concrete volatile objects suspended in the psyche. With this the individual's sensitivity to stressful events heightens and the risk of violence in a desperate attempt to rid the psyche of psychic pain is increased. Hyatt-Williams applies this theory specifically to the dynamics of murder which we shall consider further in Chapter 5.

A number of other authors have linked violent acting out to issues of loss and problems with the mourning process (Bluglass, 1990; Sohn, 1995; Zulueta, 1993). Loss here relates not only to the object, but also to the self. Trauma damages the self, leaving it changed in some way. Violence related to loss and problems with mourning is therefore fundamentally related to experiences of loss of parts of the self.

It is well known that trauma forces the personality into a state of dissociation. It leaves the self or ego vulnerable and hypersensitive to external stimuli causing extreme defensive measures, such as violence, to be taken in reaction to relatively benign events. In such cases trauma is internalized and perpetuated internally as part of a paranoid-schizoid solution. As a result no mourning or reparation of internal objects and self-representations can occur. Symington (1996) refers to a similar process where trauma is aligned with an archaic superego that constantly attacks creative and developing parts of the mind.

Whether some degree of trauma or brutalization of the self is needed to increase the individual's propensity for violence is still a debatable issue. Certainly some, like Zulueta (1993), are emphatic about the role of trauma in precipitating violence. But evidence does not always support this. In many cases trauma may not lead to future violence, nor is it the case that all violent offenders show signs of trauma. Simply isolating trauma as an indicator for the prediction of violence does not do justice to the complexity of the problem. Whether past victimization or trauma is a key factor in certain types of violence depends on how these events are internalized, other psychic resources available, and the way defences constellate around the intrapsychic manifestations of such events.

In other words, other dimensions are needed to grasp the range of possibilities here that amount to considering the 'total situation' that surrounds the traumatic happening. This would include factors like the availability of supportive others, general environmental factors and the nature of the internal world at the time. Too often the traumatic incident is taken to be a concrete object in itself and is assumed to have invariable traumatic implications. This often leads to blanket assumptions about trauma being the reason for aberrant behaviour or psychopathology. Such thoughts also lead to fixed ideas about appropriate interventions in dealing with traumatized patients where the variable and dynamic consequences of trauma are not fully considered. If these are duly considered the implications of trauma are best conceptualized in terms of an ongoing 'traumatizing process' (Cartwright and Cassidy, 2002).

I hope to show later that when trauma is evident in the rage offender it is internalized within a particular context that leads to the formation of a dangerous bad-object system that adopts particular defensive measures. As we shall see, however, this does not always emerge through exposure to trauma.

Although the implications of trauma are said to be variable, it does appear that in some cases, particularly where gross sadistic acts of violence are used, there are consistent signs that the offender has been subjected to severe cruelty and humiliation in childhood. I recall one such case, the case of Mark, that disturbed me greatly because of the heinous nature of the crimes he had committed. Mark was serving a life-sentence for four separate murders, although he confessed to many others during our interviews. On one occasion he described how he took great pleasure in forcing an unsuspecting couple to have sex in front of him before he savagely gouged out their eyes and then dumped them in the centre of town naked, in an attempt to humiliate them further. In cases like this it is not difficult to discern a great deal of hatred and disturbance in the offenders' general approach. Aggressive intentions and violence are usually easily observable as it becomes the most effective means of communication and expression. In most cases like this a history of severe victimization and cruelty is easily found. Mark, for instance, had been considerably brutalized by his father over a long period of time. He was often tied up, often forced to have sex with his sister, often forced to eat his own excrement.

In many cases, however, the link to trauma is not so simple. As Gilligan (1996) explains, trauma is not caused only by witnessing or being victim to a violent act. Words can do just as much damage to the self, in turn, causing greater vulnerability to becoming violent. As he puts it, 'Words alone can shame and reject, insult and humiliate, dishonor and disgrace, tear down self-esteem, and murder the soul' (p.49). Violence also sometimes has stronger links to other determinants or dimensions. As mentioned earlier, more subtle parental interactions leading to a diminished representational capacity may better explain why some forms of violence emerge.

Still further, Shengold (1999), in expressing how little we know about violence, observes that not all violent individuals have a traumatic or spoiling parental presence in their histories. He is convinced that violence is often a result of over-gratification or over-stimulation. Although agreeing that rage is a reaction to narcissistic injury, Shengold emphasizes the role of over-stimulation as 'the basic danger situation' (p.110). Over-stimulation creates primitive and illusive narcissistic desires for 'everything' that give rise to intense affective states. When this intensity leads to 'nothingness', however, it is easily transformed into murderous rage. The more this archaic grandiosity is over-stimulated, the further the individual has to fall when this delusion is shattered in some way. Thus, 'over-stimulation threatens annihilation and enhances ('feeds') the aggressive drive' (p.111).

Shengold also finds that parents who are afraid of their own anger cope by being over-indulgent in their parenting. The experience of anger then becomes associated with a dangerous unknown experience. Here, over-indulgence leads to these individuals having 'deficiencies in internalizing the necessary "no" in relation to their impulses and are therefore terrified of them and of their unchecked rage at inevitable frustrations' (p.xvii).

From another perspective, Hering (1997) also questions the simplistic notion of the cycle of abuse. He argues that reliance on the trauma hypothesis leads to an underestimation of our own intrinsic destructiveness and also negates the potency of violent phantasies that are not the result of abuse but lead to destructive scenarios. Certainly the 'cycle of violence theory' also cannot, without considering other intrapsychic dimensions, account for why more men engage in violence when clearly women sustain a lot more trauma and abuse.

Sexuality

What role does sexuality play in fostering violent behaviour? There are many theories about the sexual or libidinal development of the child available to us, ranging from Freud's instinctual model to Fairbairn's object-driven model. These two models perhaps represent polar opposites within psychoanalytic thinking as regards the sexual and aggressive nature of development. We have considered these in the previous chapter.

Much has been written about the fine line between sex and violence, from cases of rape, to sado-masochistic sexual practices, to serial murders. Here, a fusion of excitation, omnipotence and destructiveness can be clearly observed pointing to a preoedipal fixation or regression where differentiation between object, self, and their corresponding affects, are not apparent.

When problems with preoedipal modes of generating experience are most evident, consistent with difficulties in breaking away from the primary object, a sense of separateness and separate sexual experience is difficult to assimilate. In these cases more primitive forms of sexuality are evident where the body becomes overwhelmed by sensations that cannot be mentally represented. Sexual excitement or sensation is thus very generalized and fuses with other affects or inchoate object- and self-representations. Joseph (1997) reminds us of an important distinction to be made between mature sexuality and sexualization. Mature forms of sexuality are characterized by a rich exchange with the object leading to creativity and growth. Sexualization, on the other hand, essentially refers to the eroticization of parts of the body or mind preventing them from performing their suitable functions. It stands in the way of thinking and serves as a defence against mature object relating and painful experience.

In sadistic or perverse violence primitive forms of sexuality are used in the service of violence itself. Here, painful experience itself is sexualized, making it exciting, compelling the individual to commit such an act of violence. I briefly alluded to such a case, the case of Mark, in the previous section where acts of sex and violence were combined for the purpose of brutal humiliation and extreme suffering. In this instance Mark did not kill his victims because that would have ended their suffering and defeated his aim. In his brutal words he said once, 'I wanted to sit back and watch them squirm in pain.'

Although underlying theoretical principles have been developed considerably since Freud, the dynamics believed to be behind sadistic violence have changed little since his second revision of the term (Freud, 1920). Here sadism is viewed as being the result of destructive tendencies towards the self that have been sexualized or libidinized before being projected outwards. Generally it is agreed that those who seek violence due to exciting sexual stimulation are dominated by preoedipal experience which forms the basis of particular character or personality disorders (Biven, 1997; Fonagy and Target, 1996; Kernberg, 1984, 1992; Meloy, 1992). Once again, how this is acted out, or whether such an internal situation will lead to violence, further depends on other intrapsychic factors being considered here. As discussed earlier, however, this does not mean that oedipal conflicts and associated problems are absent in such individuals as is often inferred.

But not all preoedipal violence can be simply related to uncontained sexual excitation. Much of the recent work focusing on preoedipal dyadic themes in violent behaviour emphasizes the defensive origins of violence at this level, focusing more on the structural aspects of the psyche that make the individual vulnerable to violence. As mentioned earlier, it is generally agreed that defensive violence has its roots in attempts to ward off perceived dangers from destroying an already fragile self. In some of these cases, sensation and primitive sexual excitement are, in themselves, felt to be dangerous. Rather than this kind of violence emanating from a defined sexual part of the self, violence aims to keep sexually exciting objects and sensations away. Put another way, it forms a part of the defensive system that aims to negate libidinous activity. We shall say more about defensive systems as a separate dimension.

If we accept that sexual development is an important dimension of violence, are we able to distinguish between preoedipal and oedipal modes of experience and the propensity for violence? Related to this, can we distinguish the type of violence that occurs in relation to psychic development and sexuality?

I have already pointed out that a simple developmental distinction between oedipal and preoedipal positions is problematic. Often, preoedipal dynamics are equated with greater severity of distress, 'worse' forms of psychopathology, or, in this case, more destructive types of violence. Such a conceptualization also implies that individuals whose psychic world is dominated by whole-object experience and full genital sexuality are less capable of violence. This is not always the case. It is rather that the kind of violence displayed (its motivating factors and precipitating core conflicts) shifts depending on the individual's area of vulnerability. Further, I think a more fundamental question to ask here concerns the level at which such conflicts are represented in the psyche and the extent to which the individual is able to contain, represent, or sublimate his or her own sexual experience.[1] It can be said, however, that the potential for violence exists at all levels of sexual development, it is the nature of the violence that changes.

We have already considered two possible formulations regarding the preoedipal nature of violence where either sexual aggression or a schizoid split away from all sensate excitation dominates sexuality. It is also thought that violence that erupts as a cathartic release can often be located at the anal level of development (Abraham, 1927; Schafer, 1976; Shengold, 1991). The oedipal level, on the other hand, is mediated by representations manifesting in experiences such as rivalry, power, revenge, jealousy or competitiveness. Clearly many violent acts may be initiated at this level. Patricide, matricide, violence against authority figures or threatening groups, a brawl between men, a fight between siblings: all clearly show oedipal themes. But do these themes elicit violence themselves, or do they initiate a regression to a more primitive level of the personality that 'acts out' violently? The latter appears to be the most favoured assumption in explaining both explosive and sexual violence (Hyatt-Williams, 1998).

Oedipal conflicts and their fundamental links to sexuality, however, can elicit violence without regression. Thus violence may not always mean the collapse of mature sexual development. Indeed, many of our cultural stereotypes about the 'macho' male support the image of a powerful dominant male, implicitly condoning violence as a means to power. In this sense the Oedipus Complex remains a central organizing principle around which the image of the violent male is formed (Jukes, 1993; 1994; Person, 1993b). As Jukes (1993) points out, there is no doubt that trauma and attachment problems can be important precipitants of violence, but they cannot explain why all forms of violence are found to be far more prevalent amongst men. If the Oedipus Complex did not have such an influence, and male violence is not simplistically explained as being innate, then one would expect to have a greater proportion of violent women, as they are the more victimized sex.

Violence can occur in the service of the ego to defend and maintain a coherent sense of identity of which gender and sexuality are an important part. From the male point of view this might be seen as an attempt to uphold 'phallic power' and

---

1   Representational capacity is seen here as a separate dimension and does not necessarily go hand-in-hand with oedipal object relations as is often implied.

excessive control, or an oedipal defence against helplessness and regression to an encapsulated psychosis (Jukes, 1993). It could be argued that powerful rationalizations fostered by internal and societal factors around masculinity also encourage violence at this level without the need for regression. 'Fight and be brave like a man' or 'You are a coward for not fighting', express some of the sanctioned societal or cultural cues to violence at this level.

The role of phantasy/fantasy

Perelberg (1995b) places great importance on the instigating function of phantasy in violent behaviour when she says, 'I suggest that the key to the distinction between aggression and violence is the phantasy attached to the act and not the act itself' (p.113). The act, she claims, always comes with an underlying motive or unconscious narrative. Similarly, Hyatt-Williams (1998), referring specifically to murder, emphasizes the importance of phantasy:

> Murder occurs concretely in most cases when it has been committed many times previously in daydreams, nightmares, and sometimes in unconscious fantasy that has never become conscious.
>
> (Hyatt-Williams, 1998, p.155)

A number of important questions require consideration here, some of which have received very little attention thus far: Do fantasies always precede violent action? Are different types of fantasy or phantasy being referred to here? Can particular phantasies/fantasies and corresponding defensive organizations be linked to violent actions? In what way does the violent scenario, if at all, exist in the individual's mind prior to the act? Are enacted 'violent phantasies' quantitatively different from those that are not? These are important considerations in the assessment of violence, not all of which can be considered here. Although some have convincingly argued that specific phantasies can be linked to violence (Hyatt-Williams, 1996; Perelberg, 1995a), one needs to be cautious in understanding what type of violence is being referred to in each case. As we have seen earlier, there are so many different forms of violence and ways of defining it. Given this, it would be far too simplistic to assume that one particular group of phantasies could explain all types of violence.

Phantasy and fantasy

Implicit in Hyatt-Williams' (1998) above statement is a distinction between phantasy and fantasy, if one is to understand it from a Kleinian point of view (Klein, 1927; Isaacs, 1948). Hyatt-Williams does not appear to make use of the distinction himself, but does indicate that fantasy may occur at different levels of consciousness. In brief, phantasies are essentially unconscious and constitute deep structures of the mind from which all thought and behaviour emanate. Fantasy, on the other hand, refers to conscious surface mentation that serves what is assumed to be a sublimatory function. The distinction itself has more recently been discussed by Hinshelwood (1997). He argues that there is little need to use one of these terms to the exclusion of the other. Though traditionally viewed as representing very different theoretical standpoints, both terms refer to different levels of psychic functioning and can be used productively together.

There is merit, I believe, in using this distinction in understanding the dynamics of violence. For instance, it is usually the case that in perverse or sadistic violence, conscious violent fantasies are clearly present and, in different ways, contribute to the conscious actions of the offender. In this case the distinction between fantasy as a sublimatory activity and unconscious phantasy collapses, and what is usually destructive, but unconscious, becomes permissible in the conscious mind. Violence that is socially sanctioned, on the other hand, is clearly worked out many times consciously, but is different in the sense that these actions do not necessarily stem from unconscious mental structures. Gang members or soldiers may fantasize many times about how they would respond when threatened or under attack, but their actions may not necessarily be linked to unconscious phantasy. Obsessional neurotics may also be plagued by fantasies of violence or murder but will never act them out as the source of the unconscious phantasy underlying these thoughts is very different. Still further, in masochistic or suicidal cases, conscious fantasies are often not consonant with unconscious mentation and rather emerge as retaliatory thoughts against psychic pain.

I shall show later that in explosive forms of violence, like rage murder, where violence is primarily motivated by volatile affect, conscious fantasies of attacking an object are often not present. If violent fantasies are present in any way, they tend to be conscious fears of being attacked, rather than being fantasies of actually attacking. This does not mean, however, that these individuals do not possess particular murderous phantasy constellations that further explain their behaviour. These brief examples hopefully demonstrate that the distinction between phantasy and fantasy holds some heuristic value in investigating the nature of violent acts.

Often phantasies, having deep structural influences on the mind, can be matched with particular defensive organizations. For example, the phantasy of annihilation of a part of the self may be matched with a defensive organization characterized by projective defences aimed at destroying parts of the self represented in other objects. However, there is not always a one-to-one match between phantasy and defence. Broadly speaking, defences may both enact or work against phantasy constellations. For this reason I have chosen to discuss the defensive system as a separate intrapsychic dimension.

Furthermore, whether phantasies are enacted or not is not solely dependent on the defensive system. The level at which phantasies are represented in the psyche is also important here. Here we need to understand phantasy alongside the capacity for representation. This relates to representational capacity referred to earlier. For instance, Hering (1997) suggests that destructive parts of the personality are fuelled by what he calls a 'concrete dream'. Here phantasy cannot occur in a symbolized form and therefore can only be externalized in a concrete form. It exists as a frozen phantasy that has eluded any elaboration or influence by both internal and external forces. Hopefully this again illustrates the need for a multi-dimensional approach to understanding the outbreak of violence. I now turn to considering the content of fantasies/phantasies related to violence.

Content of phantasy/fantasy

Although Freud did not discuss the conceptual distinctions between violence and aggression, Perelberg (1995b) argues, in a thorough analysis of his use of the term, that he consistently related violence to phantasies of the primal scene and the Oedipus Complex. Freud, she argues, related violence to key aspects of myths of our own origins. Notably, the parental sexual act is experienced by children as violent on the father's part and it is here that the phantasy of murderousness towards the penetrating father is at its height. Further, phantasies related to the idea that sons would kill their fathers in order to have intercourse with their mothers also leads Perelberg to the conclusion that violence, on Freud's part, is linked to unconscious phantasies of this nature.

Following Freud's emphasis on the oedipal origins of the neuroses, many of the earlier writings on violence and murder appear to emphasize oedipal phantasies as being prominent in acts of violence. Menninger, for instance, understood some forms of aggression and destructiveness as being connected to castrating or muti-lating phantasies originally directed at parents. Others have argued that violent encounters have their roots in fearful phantasies of sexual inadequacy that expose the individual in a shameful way (Abrahamsen, 1973; Bromberg, 1961).

Perelberg's analysis of violent patients supports the idea that the primal scene is an important core phantasy in considering violence. She expands on Freud's original ideas, however, by emphasizing the relationship with the preoedipal mother as important. This follows a general trend in psychoanalytic thinking where the influence of the first 2 years of life and the maternal relationship are given more emphasis. Recent understandings of the violent patient are no excep-tion.

There appears to be common agreement that self-preservative forms of violence are often accompanied by phantasies of feeling engulfed or attacked by the maternal object (Bergaret, 1984; Kernberg, 1984; Perelberg, 1995b; Shengold, 1989; Sohn, 1995). Congruent with the symbiotic maternal object relations dis-cussed earlier, some have found that phantasies underlying violence depict a dilemma between fusion and a desperate desire for separateness. Glasser (1998) argues that this points to 'a core complex' that is present in all of us but underlies all violent behaviour when tampered with or left unresolved. The complex is expressed in phantasies of longing for fusion and union with the object, whilst at the same time, fearing being merged and as a consequence, annihilated by the object.

Biven (1977) reports on a similar dilemma in his analysis of an adolescent boy who had undergone severe deprivation as an infant and was from a violent home. The core phantasy manifested itself in the child's thoughts of being 'enveloped' by skin. Biven explains his interpretation of 'envelopment' as follows:

> The aim of such envelopment would not simply be reunion with the primary love object, but borrowing as it were, the strength and cohesiveness from a more powerful object ... in other words the skin served as a concrete part object of another's strength.
>
> (Biven, 1977, p.351)

It is a phantasy of incorporation with the effect of having access to the mother's strength and containment. He considers the meaning of this further, claiming that the consequent retardation in superego development in this case prevented resolution of the parental relationship. As a result, the child lived in constant search for new love objects to fulfil this phantasy with violence erupting if this was threatened in any way. The phantasy here is thus a defence against aggressive impulses originally aimed at a mother who is experienced as mad and murderous.

Others have seen violence as stemming from a phantasied attack on the body of the mother (Bateman, 1999; Campbell, 1999; Fonagy and Target, 1995). In some cases the mother's body is the target of violence as she is experienced as being in possession of her patient's bodily, affective and intellectual functioning. The central underlying phantasy appears to be about a violent engulfing experience where a violent response attempts to create a space for a separate existence. It is characterized by a particular kind of paranoid-schizoid experience fuelled by the phantasy that the individual was conceived out of a violent interchange with the mother with no conception of a paternal object present. The central structuring phantasy is one of feeling consumed by unmanageable, indigestible experience with no relief or containment apparent.

This is central to Hyatt-Williams' (1998) ideas as to why self-preservative acts of violence occur. The individual becomes consumed by evacuative and annihilatory phantasies aimed primarily at escaping a more 'deathly' experience by defensively attacking it. There appears to be general agreement about this being a defining feature of this kind of violence. Hyatt-Williams, in particular, emphasizes a link between evacuation and phantasies of violence that have, at their core, indigestible experience or fantasies of death or trauma. We shall consider his ideas further in exploring different formulations of rage-type murder in Chapter 5.

Most of the above pertains to defensive acts of violence. In sadistic forms of violence, fantasies of violence are not only conscious and well developed, but are also characteristically tinged with sexual excitation. Although preoedipal themes, particularly of engulfment and fusion, do appear to characterize these forms of violence, it is the role they play as part of a perverse creative act that appears particularly different about the fantasies of such offenders.

In an exploratory study of a serial killer, Biven (1997) argues that, although often obscured, a process of dehumanization is always evident in this form of violence. The central phantasy constellation forms around a repetitive need to obliterate all humanness in the self and the object which is accompanied by intense sexual arousal. It becomes an attempt to freeze experience in a 'tableau' of his own perverse creations that are repeatedly destroyed in order to be re-created. He describes this repetition perpetuated by phantasy as follows:

> The impotent, terrified child becomes the potent but detached adult man acting a part in a play that he can barely fathom. Yet he is always dissatisfied. Each enactment of the fragmented past becomes less and less representative or connected to the human world. Such a man is not content with a dead mother or a headless eviscerated mother. What he wants is the total disappearance and reappearance of mother. But, as we can see, mother's disappearance is not simply a wish that she would go away. In fact, one could argue that in the repetitious and compulsive enactment, the serial killer is constantly bringing her back to life, only to kill her again and again.
>
> (Biven, 1997, p.40)

Here conscious fantasy is partly an attempt to hide childhood trauma behind a 'grotesque, childish collage of fact and feeling, distortion and desire' (p.44), and partly a re-enactment of the trauma. As we have seen earlier, although plagued by these fantasies, such individuals seldom show any understanding of their meaning.

Discussing a similar case, Harris and Pontius (1975) argue that acts of dismemberment are perpetuated by fantasies aimed at a purposeful disintegration of the object in order 'to reconstitute it in a subjectively more meaningful way' (p.7). The fantasy here manifests as a primitive reinstatement of a primary identification or fusion with an omnipotent and gratifying object which can then be incorporated into the self.

Whether there are qualitative differences in fantasy/phantasy constellations when it comes to defining their level of dangerousness in terms of leading to actual physical violence or not still remains to be explored. Clearly, we know that the level of dangerousness expressed in fantasy is dependent on considering a number of other internal factors, such as whether the fantasy is ego-syntonic or not. But are there differences in the way fantasies are expressed, their chronicity and their content that can be related to the degree of dangerousness. A lot more work is needed in this area if we are to use this dimension productively to assess violent patients or use it to give an indication of the propensity towards violence. Here I have simply attempted to show that broad differences between manifestations of the fantasy/phantasy distinction, as well as possible differences in content, do exist in different forms of violence.

Defensive organizations

One might argue that although all the above dimensions are important to our understanding of violence, the ability to inhibit violence is essentially dependent on the nature and strength of the defensive system. Although this may be correct, it still remains to ask, as Shengold (1999) does, 'How and why does an inadequacy of defence against the discharge of violent impulses arise?' (p.xvi). Here we are reliant on other dimensions of violence to assist us in our understanding. The nature of internal object relations, accompanying phantasies and external stressors, all influence the defensive system's action at that moment when violence may potentially occur.

Many different kinds of defensive manoeuvres have been associated with violent acts. Perhaps the most common formulation regarding violence and defence is that it represents a collapse of the psychological defensive system where the individual is left with only action (Biven, 1977; Hyatt-Williams, 1998; Lefer, 1984; Menninger *et al.*, 1963). According to Hitchcock (1996), for instance, violence erupts when mechanisms of displacement are weakened causing the individual's ego to be overwhelmed with an unmanageable affective state. Using Anna Freud's words, he calls this anticipatory state of violence the 'dread of the strength of the instincts' (p.102). This is similar to the violent acts discussed by Menninger where 'episodic dyscontrol', a rupturing in the ego, leads to violence.

As mentioned earlier, violence has also been formulated as a means of identifying with the aggressor (Zulueta, 1993). From another perspective, Treurniet (1996) and Symington (1996) view some forms of violence as an ultimate defence against intolerable guilt. Others have argued that it acts as a defensive means of maintaining attachments (Bowlby, 1969) or maintaining contiguous contact with the object (Biven, 1977). Still further, violence has also been understood to function as a means of defensively ridding the self of toxic mental states (Hyatt-Williams, 1998; Sohn, 1995). Related to this, from an interactive point of view, it is seen as a defence against further violence or pain being directed at the self.

The above are but a few of the many possible formulations. The aim here is to consider the broader issues of how defences might be used in violent behaviour. What the above possibilities illustrate, however, is that it is not always the case that defences aim to inhibit the aggression. They themselves may also lead to violence. Violence may well be incorporated into the defences as a means of protection and/or persecution.

One way of explaining these differences is to separate repression as a primary defence from more primitive interactional defences (Bateman, 1996). Repression essentially functions as an internal defence keeping forbidden impulses in check. If this fails the ego is flooded by impulses that may lead to violence. The phenomenological experience of erupting into a violent rage is often depicted as a collapse of an internal repressive force.

On the other hand, more primitive defences, such as splitting and projective identification, which have appropriately been termed the 'action defences' (Lecours and Bouchard, 1997), incorporate violence as a means of defence. Violence may be used here as a paranoid means of warding off attacking objects or as a means of attempting to rid the self of intolerable mental states.

It is usually a system of defences, however, that work together as opposed to a single defensive manoeuvre that leads to violence. Here the Kleinian understanding of defensive or pathological organizations is most useful. The term 'pathological organization' (Steiner, 1982), emerged from the work of Kleinian analysts interested in understanding borderline and narcissistic personality organizations. It refers to a system of defences and object relations that work, or lock, together so as to avoid psychic pain and to effect a deadening stasis in the emotional life of the individual. Because the defences form a system, this aspect of the personality becomes extremely resistant to change. O'Shaughnessy (1981) explains the difference between what she understands as normal defences and what she calls 'defensive organizations': 'Unlike defences – piecemeal, transient to a greater or lesser extent, recurrent – which are a normal part of development, a defensive organization is a fixation, a pathological formation' (p.363). Whereas defences, she goes on to say, form part of working through paranoid and depressive anxieties, defensive organizations shut down the personality to any experience of disturbance.

In reviewing this development in the Kleinian school, Spillius (1988) identifies two central aspects of defensive organizations that have emerged in the literature: First, pathological organizations have been used to describe a system that includes internal objects, phantasies and impulses existing between the paranoid-schizoid and depressive positions. Second, pathological organizations stem from the dominance of the 'bad self' over the rest of the personality. These organizations have their roots in more aggressive aspects of the individual which may be used in a number of different ways to avoid emotional growth.

Borderline and narcissistic defensive organizations are often found to be present in violent individuals across different categories of violence (Gacono, 1990; Gallwey, 1985; Hyatt-Williams, 1998; Kernberg, 1992; Meloy, 1992). The battery of defences being referred to here are primitive defences such as splitting, denial, idealization, devaluation and projective identification. As well as these individual defences contributing to a violent mental state, there appear to be a number of important factors that lead to physical destructiveness becoming a part of the defensive organization.

First, the way in which internal objects lock together to form a rigid and inflexible defensive system goes some way in explaining why some parts of the personality remain aggressive in nature and unarticulated by experience. The system serves as a barrier to unwanted experience and entrenches a split in the personality. Because of the static and inflexible nature of the system, sudden unexpected shifts in the psyche immobilize the defences and release encapsulated violent affects and object constellations.

Bateman (1999) found this to be the case in exploring violence in narcissistic states. He adopts Rosenfeld's (1987) distinction between 'thin' and 'thick-skinned' narcissistic states in an attempt to understand violent action. He argues that violence is most likely to occur when a shift between these two rigid defensive patterns take place. In a similar way, Hyatt-Williams (1998) argues that flight into action is precipitated by a rapid shift from the depressive position to the paranoid-schizoid position where persecutory anxiety predominates and threatens the ability to contain.

The rigid barrier that characterizes these kinds of defensive organization might, in some cases, be difficult to distinguish from repression. Both keep parts of the psyche away from reality or consciousness. They have very different functions, however. Repression, a more mature defence, aims to push down what is forbidden or detrimental to realistic development. The defensive system, on the other hand, aims to prevent learning from experience and any consequent emotional growth by splitting off parts and functions of the personality.

Thus the splitting of the personality in this way has been found to be an important second factor in the defensive functioning of the violent individual. From different perspectives, Winnicott (1965) understands the origins of antisocial acts to be in a split between the False and True self. Glasser (1997) explores 'simulation' as a key defence against development of the real self, whilst Gallwey (1985) considers the role of the 'pseudo-personality' in violent criminals. These formulations bear some similarity to the defensive system that appears to be prevalent in rage-type offenders – what I have termed the 'narcissistic exoskeleton' (Cartwright, 2002). We shall return to explore the detail of this structure in Chapter 6.

The degree to which the defensive system is characterized by paranoid or psychotic splitting that threatens the individual's hold on reality is an important factor to consider here. In this state the self is vulnerable and over-reacts to benign stimuli. A violent outcome is also more likely when there is an intolerance of any depressive experience. In these cases the experience of loss or ambivalence cannot be held in mind and is evacuated via projective identification. Here violence is used as an immediate solution to ending the painful experience through annihilating it in the object it is projected into.

On the other hand, Sohn (1995) found, in working with particularly disturbed patients who had committed unprovoked assaults, that violence can also result from a failure to use projective identification. He claims that projective identification could not be used as a means of ridding the self of frightening psychic elements because of the concrete nature of internal objects. Here, the concretization of objects served to enable the patients to keep objects inside themselves, avoiding the dread of an empty mind. The action of projective identification is thus felt to be a devastating loss, as opposed to it being a vehicle for evacuation and relief. If such patients could put it into words, Sohn argues, they would say: 'I can't project the experience of loss – if I did I would empty my mind and myself completely' (p.574).

Finally, the action of projective identification, viewed from an interactive perspective, also offers an explanation as to why aggression may escalate into violence. Used in this way, the concept transcends a difficult conceptual divide between intrapsychic and interpersonal processes. Once the intolerable psychic state has been projected, the recipient may himself experience it as intolerable and return it along with his own defensive anger. This in turn leads to a more uncontainable psychic state that becomes impossible to metabolize by, or between, the individuals involved. An insult that leads to an argument and then to violence is a broad example of this kind of interaction. Here victim, perpetrator and specific aspects of the context become part of a dangerous juggling act where undigested emotional states are irresolvably passed between perpetrator and victim. The situation becomes entrapping with neither party being able to opt out, or contain, the projected state. As a result, an escalating violent situation ensues. This kind of understanding moves towards viewing violence not simply in terms of the perpetrator, but in terms of the total situation. Ideas in this area may contribute a great deal to understanding interpersonal conflict and violence but have yet to be fully developed in the area of applied psychoanalysis.

Interaction with the external situation

> [A] violent act is always a triangle. A study of one person can never explain it. Nor a study of two. We always have to visualize the potential influence on one another of first, the perpetrator; second, the victim; third; the reaction of the other people in the smaller or wider circle.
>
> (Wertham, 1962, p.42)

I turn now to the last intrapsychic dimension of violence to be considered. Although I am essentially concerned with the internal world of the violent offender, this of course cannot be studied in complete isolation from events evident in the external situation at the time of the violent act. Of importance here is the interface between the intrapsychic and the external situation. All too often this is ignored as a key factor leading to criticisms regarding the solipsistic nature of psychoanalysis. Perhaps this is due to the fact that in the therapeutic setting most external factors are held constant and emphasis is placed on internal experience. In the analysis of behaviours that occur outside of the therapeutic setting, however, external factors cannot be ignored. This is especially the case in studying violence where a majority of violent acts can be shown to have external precipitants, no matter how benign in themselves. I view the interface as occurring from both directions: First, it relates to how the external circumstances impact on the individual, in turn, altering his or her internal world. Second, studying external factors helps us understand how the individual manipulates external objects to fulfil an internal purpose.

It is common knowledge that the external situation has an important role to play in weakening defences and prompting regressions. Often external situations associated with a difficult past situation weaken the individual's displacement mechanisms, leaving him feeling overwhelmed by the situation. Indeed, sometimes simply the build-up of external factors that cannot be mastered or controlled may precipitate violence. Hyatt-Williams (1998) describes this type of violent situation as occurring when 'too much happens too soon'. Fromm (1973) takes this point to the extreme by arguing that destructive aggression or violence is 'not due to a greater aggressive potential but to the fact of aggression-producing conditions' (p.185).

Does this mean that we are all capable of violence of some kind when the pressure gets too much? This, of course, is dependent on individual vulnerabilities expressed in the different dimensions outlined above. It would also depend, however, on the nature of the external factors themselves. Clearly severe trauma or an extremely threatening situation would propel many into using violence defensively as a last resort. Milder provocations, on the other hand, would cause a wide range of reactions and would depend more on intrapsychic factors.

We also need to consider 'condoning' external factors, as opposed to provocative or instigating events, that influence violent action. These are factors, immediate or enduring, that facilitate 'acceptable' forms of violence. The most obvious example here is the violence committed during war. External influences are internalized in an ego-syntonic way and differ greatly in their intrapsychic influence.

The external situation – particularly the crime scene and antecedent events – also requires thorough investigation as its nature sheds light on the degree to which pathological states contribute to the violent act. Pathological states can be assumed to play more of a part in violent acts when there is little provocation from the environment. Here, external factors serve more of a representational role, giving us clues about the individual's internal world. This includes, for instance, the way the offender, consciously or unconsciously, creates the crime scene, interacts with the victim or makes a weapon available. Biven's (1997) attempt at understanding the internal world of a serial killer provides a good example of this process. These factors, however, also remain important in less glamorous or perverse forms of violence. The events that lead the offender into a potentially violent situation, for example, may say a lot about his or her unconscious motivations. Precipitating external events may also give us clues as to how the victim features in the internal world of the offender. This has important implications for working out whether the offender will attack a wide range of individuals or only a small target pool of people who hold a particular representational meaning for the individual. Such factors are important when assessing the dangerousness of the individual.

The victim, being part of the external situation, also makes different impressions on the offender's internal world. Those who have attempted to explore the victim's role in acts of violence have tended to consider only their intrapsychic motivations. For example, how unconscious guilt may motivate an individual to seek punishment unconsciously (Abrahamsen, 1973; Goreta, 1995). To continue with this example, whilst this is important, it tends to underestimate the interactional nature of the psychological system. The individual may seek an unconscious form of punishment but this is always in interaction with an external object. In this sense, the victim's role in manipulating the interpersonal situation towards a violent outcome is central. The same victim, for instance, may constantly put him- or herself in a situation where he or she compulsively insults or picks pointless arguments with others, hence manipulating his or her objects into a defensive attack.

In other words, seen solely from an intrapsychic perspective, the initiator of a violent act becomes the focus of our attention regarding his or her defences, projective identifications and so forth. From an interactional perspective, however, it can be seen that in some cases, the violent offender may well be on the receiving end of powerful interpersonal dynamics that can no longer be tolerated, thus causing him or her to retaliate. In short, the victim's role and the situation itself thus become important factors to consider. An example of the complexity of the interaction that might occur is reflected below in Hyatt-Williams' discussion of the projection of the 'death constellation':

> The person into whom the death constellation has been put by projective identification is felt to contain that part of the owner of the death constellation. There is also a supposition that the death constellation can be bounced back into the owner as and when the latter feels threatened. At this point, there is acute danger of a murderous attack upon the person into whom it is imagined that the death constellation has been put. Sometimes the projector reintrojects his intention, sparing his victim.
>
> (Hyatt-Williams, 1998, p.45)

Later on Hyatt-Williams returns to this theme explaining that 'after a few projective and introjective transactions the situation becomes confused and the motivation becomes more and more mixed' (p.118). This goes to show how confusing the situation between victim and offender can become where an interpersonal escalation of tension plays a key role in precipitating violence.

CONCLUDING COMMENTS

I have attempted to explore what we know currently about various forms of violence in terms of how intrapsychic processes ultimately lead to an attack on the physical world. In addition, I have used a dimensional approach to emphasize the complexity of the problem. A linear approach to defining different forms of violence does not appear adequate for our purposes here as the intrapsychic world of the individual operates at many different levels, with no one form of violence being the same as the other. Further, depending on the kind of violence, different dimensions are bound to hold relatively different explanatory powers. As well as their clinical significance in treating individuals who engage in violent behaviour, such observations also have implications for forensic investigation and the assessment of dangerousness. We shall return to these dimensions later in considering the internal world of the rage-type murderer after we have outlined key considerations in this area of investigation.

Part II

Investigating rage-type murder

Chapter 3

Defining the parameters of the act: problems and dilemmas

I begin my investigation of rage-type murder by considering some of the defining features of the act. We have already established that rage-type murder refers to a murderous act triggered by a sudden explosive affective state. We have also established that rage-type violence is best understood in psychoanalytic terms as being affective or self-preservative in nature. There are, of course, many different forms of violent crime and many different reasons why some of these result in a homicidal act. In criminological terms, murder committed as an act of rage fits the category of expressive or hostile violent crime (Weiner and Wolfgang, 1989; Salfati, 2000). Offenders belonging to this category need to be distinguished from individuals who have psychopathic, perverse or psychotic motives. They further need to be distinguished from those individuals who have committed murder in order to fulfil a criminal motive.

Rage-type murder has been reported by many to be a common form of homicidal behaviour (Abrahamsen, 1973; Bromberg, 1961; Gilligan, 1996; Hodgins, 1993; Hollin, 1989; Hyatt-Williams, 1996; Meloy, 1992; Wertham, 1937). However, there appears to be no reliable statistical enumeration available indicating how common this form of murder actually is. This is because most of the statistical studies exploring the incidence of homicide simply make a distinction between 'normal' homicide, 'abnormal' homicide and psychopathic homicide (e.g. Blackburn, 1993; Bluglass and Bowden, 1990). It is difficult to use these kinds of study in considering rage-type murder as it has not been consistently reported as belonging to one particular category. Although there has been a considerable amount of research on personality and mental illness related to violence or murder, the parameters and characteristics of the act itself still require further exploration.

With the exception of Revitch and Schlesinger (1981), Meloy (1992) and Hyatt-Williams (1998), there has been very little recent work in this area. There are, however, a number of early seminal studies that remain relevant in defining the act (Menninger et al., 1963; Ruotolo, 1968; Weiss et al., 1960; Wertham, 1937).

My understanding of the act draws on criminological, psychological and psychiatric perspectives. I am interested here in refining our understanding of the defining parameters of explosive forms of violence which, in turn, raises important questions and problems. It should be noted that, aside from some general comments regarding the psychodynamics of the act, detailed discussion on psychodynamic features will be reserved for later chapters.

The following description from my work with Simon, a 32-year-old sailor who had murdered his wife, typifies the events and situations that surround the act of rage-type murder. I have included other relevant details of the case to which I shall return in exploring contributing psychopathology and the intrapsychic nature of the event.

SIMON

Simon stabbed his wife seventeen times in a fit of rage. He had minimal recall of the incident and was taken to hospital the following morning because he had taken an overdose of tablets immediately prior to the attack.

Simon was the youngest in his family. He had a sister 2 years older than him and a brother 4 years his senior. When Simon was 4 years old his mother died from a sudden illness. A year later his father remarried but remained largely absent from the family because of work commitments. Simon and his brother and sister were largely left alone with their new mother. From the very beginning it appears that his relationship with her was difficult. He felt controlled and manipulated by her. Court proceedings made little reference to this relationship, but, from his descriptions, it appeared that it involved considerable abuse. He was forced to do work around the house for extended hours and was never allowed visits from friends. He also recalled his stepmother depriving him of food when she was not happy with his behaviour.

Simon spoke about his 'real mother' as being 'a true providing mother'. He had very little memory of this, but claimed that he 'felt it in the way [he] knew that no-one else had been able to care the way she did'. His feelings towards his stepmother were very different. He recalled incidents that gave the impression that he still felt persecuted by her. One such incident that appeared to stick in his mind involved him having to stay up late at night to clean floors when he desperately wanted to go and sleep. Interestingly, he often spoke of these incidents in the present tense.

Immediately after finishing school Simon made a decision to go into the navy based solely on his need to get away from, in his view, a domineering and controlling stepmother. Although his job involved very little sea travel, after leaving he had very little contact with his father or stepmother. For the first 6 years, before he was married, he had no contact with them at all.

In reaction to his past, Simon implied that he had created a 'private part' of himself that was always thinking about ways of 'escaping' and dreaming of 'doing great things'. This part of him felt 'adult' and was associated with a need to protect vulnerable things around him. His father was felt to be inaccessible and complacent in dealing with any of the difficulties at home and, as a result, he was seen to be allied with his stepmother's motives. Simon was clearly ashamed of the way he and his siblings were treated and made every effort to hide this part of his life from others. 'I wanted to turn my back on the whole embarrassment', he recalled once. Often he would hide away from others, or stay away from school, to keep himself from a pending sense of 'embarrassment' that he claimed to experience regularly.

His thoughts of being a sailor were strongly related to the achievement of becoming an adequate man. There was a clear sense of him feeling that he had to do a lot more than other men to 'measure up', but in the end he 'achieved great things'. His achievements here followed a distinct pattern where he prided himself in constantly offering his services in an over-obliging manner to other officers whom he idealized. Simon had a history of avoiding assertive action as it was associated with aggression. He particularly went out of his way to avoid aggressive encounters in the navy. He did so by placating others as soon as there were any signs of this occurring.

After two short relationships, Simon married and had one child. He paid for an elaborate wedding himself and saw it as an opportunity to show what he could provide for his wife. He only invited his father to his wedding; his stepmother was excluded. 'With never having had any love', he claimed, referring to his wife, 'I knew I had to make this bond very strong.' Simon spoke of his wife in idealized terms as if nothing negative ever happened. If it did, it was quickly 'forgotten about' and was associated with him needing to do more to build on their relationship.

After 2 years of marriage Simon discovered that his wife had been having a love affair with another man. At the time, Simon ostensibly 'forgave' her and the event appeared to have caused very little conflict in their marriage. He did not, however, discuss it openly with his wife. He responded, in a rather elaborate way, by trying to pay her more attention, ensuring that she had everything she needed. A few months later a friend told him that this wife was still having an affair. The same scenario followed, with him forgiving her and trying to make things better. However, a short while later, his wife asked for a separation as she felt that the relationship was not able to fulfil her needs. After hearing that his wife was leaving him Simon had become notably withdrawn and depressed.

A few weeks later, however, Simon's wife invited him to visit her with a view to 'trying to work things out and get back together'. Despite feeling depressed, Simon claimed that he had managed to recover somewhat and had started moving in a different circle of friends. He felt that he knew that his wife 'would eventually come to her senses'. He recalled feeling very good about this because he felt his 'positivity had rubbed off on her' and that is why she now wanted him back.

He arrived that Saturday night and spent some time playing with his daughter outside before entering the house to greet his wife. After putting his daughter to bed, they began cordially discussing recent events and sat down together to eat dinner like 'old times', something he had suggested they do. During the meal his wife began to talk about 'her new life', where she wanted to live, and the possibility of a new job. It was at this point that Simon remembered beginning to feel upset again by the situation and found himself becoming overwhelmed with anger as she spoke.

He remembered them beginning to argue about her affair and how he kept on saying that he 'just wanted to forget about it and carry on' with their lives together. She too became angry and wished out loud that he would 'just disappear and die'. Promptly after this he took an overdose of pills and immediately attacked her with a knife.

From this point on, he had very little recall of the events that followed. He remembered a knife and 'rolling around the floor with a knife', but he felt as if he was 'doing nothing with it'. He remembered seeing his wife on the kitchen floor with multiple stab wounds all over her body. He remembered the blood and calling the police, but little else.

Simon had no previous history of violent or aggressive behaviour towards anyone and claimed never to have thought of killing his wife. The only conscious fantasies he recalled were related to the distress he felt about her leaving him. No history of psychological signs or symptoms of distress were reported as occurring prior to the build-up to the murder. He described the murder as leaving him with a sense that 'something took her'; he could not believe that he had done such a thing. He could only understand it as 'something inside me snapping ... something happened *to* me', a subtle means of separating himself from being the perpetrator of such a crime.

The medical report indicated that multiple deep stab wounds to the body killed his wife. The knife he used was an ordinary kitchen knife.

DEFINING FEATURES OF THE ACT

Along with the overwhelming rage that precipitated Simon's actions, there are a number of other characteristics immediately evident here that set this kind of murder apart from other homicides. Most notably, it appears to be out of character, there is no clear apparent motive for the murder and the act is not premeditated in any way.

A number of other terms have been used to describe this kind of murder, each one tending to focus on one of the above characteristics. Blackman *et al.* (1963), Lamberti *et al.* (1958) and Weiss *et al.* (1960), all part of the same research group at Washington University, use the term 'sudden murder' to emphasize the peculiar nature of the murderous act. 'Sudden' refers not only to the impulsiveness of the act itself, but also to its being an isolated event uncharacteristic of the individual's usual behaviour. They describe the act as being committed by:

> a person who, without having been involved in any previous serious aggressive antisocial acts, suddenly, unlawfully, and intentionally kills (or makes a serious attempt to kill) another human being. The murder is 'sudden' in the sense that it appears to be a single, isolated, unexpected episode of violent,

impulsive acting-out behaviour – behaviour which is never well thought out, behaviour which has no obvious purpose or hope for personal advantage or profit foreseeable as a result.

(Weiss *et al.*, 1960, p.669)

Other terms that have been used to describe a similar form of homicide include motiveless murder (Satten *et al.*, 1960; Sohn, 1995; Stone, 1993), dissociative murder (Tanay, 1969), affective murder (Meloy, 1988), explosive murder (Bromberg, 1961; Menninger *et al.*, 1963), and catathymic murder (Meloy, 1992; Wertham, 1937) .

There are two possible clinical disorders worth considering, related to the act itself, when one uses *The Diagnostic and Statistical Manual of Mental Disorders IV* (American Psychiatric Association, 1994): Intermittent Explosive Disorder and Brief Psychotic Disorder. The former is defined by the following criteria:

A.   Several discrete episodes of failure to resist aggressive impulses that result in serious assaultive acts or destruction of property.
B.   The degree of aggressiveness expressed during the episodes is grossly out of proportion to any precipitating psychological stressors.
C.   The aggressive episodes are not better accounted for by another mental disorder (e.g. Antisocial personality disorder, Borderline personality disorder, a Psychotic disorder, a Manic Episode, Conduct Disorder, or Attention-Deficit/Hyperactivity Disorder) and are not due to the direct physiological effects of a substance (e.g. a drug of abuse, a medication) or a general medical condition (e.g. a head trauma, Alzheimer's disease).

(APA, 1994, p.612)[1]

There has been very little research exploring the nature of this disorder and its relationship to different types of violence. There do, however, appear to be some similarities between explosive acts of violence and what is described above. Although *The Diagnostic and Statistical Manual of Mental Disorders IV* reports that it is a relatively rare diagnosis, Felthous *et al.* (1991) report an 18.9 per cent incidence amongst violent men. They also found that most of the rage reactions occurred without a noticeable prodromal period. Although most offenders remained oriented during the outburst, a majority only had partial recollection of the event.

Although there are similarities between the diagnosis of intermittent explosive disorder and rage-type murder, one factor stands out as an exception: most of the murderers who I have worked with do not report having a history of explosive outbursts nor is there typically any other evidence of this being the case. Simon, for

1   Reprinted with permission from the *Diagnostic and Statistical Manual of Mental Disorders*, fourth edition, text revison, copyright 2000 American Pyschiatric Association.

instance, had no history of violence whatsoever between him and his wife and elsewhere. In fact, as his case shows, such offenders usually actually stay away from any behaviour that may be construed as 'aggressive'. In other words, a pattern of aggressive outbursts is not typical of the profile I have explored. I shall return to possible explanations for this later.

The other diagnosis, brief psychotic disorder, also may describe some of the clinical elements that appear in rage-type murder. It is defined by the presence of vivid psychotic symptoms, such as hallucinations and incoherence. Although not always the case, the disorder often occurs in response to a particular stressor in the individual's life. It is defined by the following criteria:

A. The presence of one (or more) of the following symptoms:

    (a) delusions
    (b) hallucinations
    (c) disorganized speech (e.g. frequent derailment or incoherence)
    (d) grossly disorganized or catatonic behavior
    Note: Do not include a symptom if it is a culturally sanctioned response pattern.

B. Duration of an episode of the disturbance is at least 1 day but less than 1 month, with eventual full return to premorbid level of functioning.

C. The disturbance is not better accounted for by a Mood Disorder With Psychotic Features, Schizoaffective Disorder, or Schizophrenia and is not due to the direct physiological effects of a substance (e.g. a drug of abuse, a medication) or a general medical condition.

                                                                   (APA, 1994, p.304)

In contrast to intermittent explosive disorder, this diagnosis requires that there be a gross break with reality where considerable disturbance of the individual's perceptual functioning occurs. Although in some cases of rage-type murder this has been reported (Menninger *et al.*, 1963; Weiss *et al.*, 1960), it appears that in most cases only minor dissociative states, by comparison, occur (Bromberg, 1961; Gilligan, 1996; Hyatt-Williams, 1998). Simon's patchy amnesia and subjective account of his rage are typical in this regard. Before the outburst, however, there are no signs of psychotic thinking or inappropriate behaviour. Further, although dissociative states may be present for some time prior to an act of violence, this is not usually the case in rage murder. Here, dissociation usually occurs along with a sudden surge of rage at the time of the murder and remits again immediately afterwards. Although there is dissociation, hallucinations do not occur. In terms of diagnosis then, although intermittent explosive disorder appears to come closer to defining the act, neither diagnosis sufficiently accounts for all clinical features. More importantly, however, the homicidal act is far more complex than any single diagnosis. The inadequacy of psychiatric diagnosis in defining disorders or syndromes related to homicidal behaviour has been noted by a number of authors (Meloy, 1992; Stone, 1993; Wertham, 1950).

In what could be considered the first attempt to outline the complexity of the act, Wertham (1937) formulated a particular sequence of clinical events that occur in the build-up to violent behaviour of this kind. He called this *the catathymic crisis*. Wertham uses the term 'catathymia', taken from Maier's (in Meloy, 1992) work in 1912 on affect-idea complexes that overwhelm conscious thought and control, to emphasize the affective nature of this process. Ultimately this leads to a conceived plan of violence and a compulsion to carry it out. It may not necessarily always result in murder, but murder is included as one of the possible consequences of the affective state. He describes the sequence of events as follows:

> A traumatic psychogenic experience precipitates an unbearable and seemingly unsolvable inner situation leading to extreme emotional tension; the subject holds the outer situation entirely responsible for this inner tension; his thinking becomes more and more ego-centric; with apparent suddenness a crystallization point is reached in the idea that a violent act against another or against himself is the only way out. After a prolonged inner struggle this violent act is attempted or carried out. It is followed immediately by an almost complete removal of the preceding emotional tension, but the patient does not gain insight at this time. There follows a superficially normal period of varying length, usually several months, after which an inner equilibrium is established, which leads to insight.
>
> (Wertham, 1937, p.796)

Later, in *Dark Legend*, a more detailed study of a single case of murder, Wertham (1950) reformulates this clinical process into a five-stage process summarized as follows: first, after an injurious precipitating experience, an inner uneasiness develops. Thinking becomes self-centred and the precipitating event is held responsible for this. Second, thoughts about a violent act being the only solution begin to occur and a consequent inner struggle develops. Third, inner tension escalates. Fourth, the violent act is carried out followed by a superficial return to normality, but with no insight into the event. Finally, this is eventually followed by the realization that the outer situation does not account for the extreme violent act that was perpetrated.

To develop this further, I shall elaborate on different aspects of Wertham's description and draw on key characteristics that have subsequently been used to define the act and its surrounding situation. I shall outline what I consider to be five key determinants central to understanding the act itself. They are: the affective nature of the act, its apparent motivelessness, the dissociative process, the distinction between chronic and acute affective reactions, and, lastly, the situational characteristics of the act.

Explosive affect

The most central defining feature of the catathymic crisis is the eruption of an overwhelming and unbearable affective state preceding the violent act or murder. Karl Menninger's research group, in the 1960s, conducted a number of studies focused on this affective form of violence. He called it 'episodic dyscontrol' in an attempt to convey, from an economic point of view, sudden lapses in ego control that would allow a surge of aggression to be acted out (Menninger, *et al.*, 1963; Menninger, 1966, 1973).

Consistent with this, reports of such incidents usually describe the act as 'unnecessarily violent' (Menninger *et al.*, 1963, p.239) where the victims have been shot or stabbed many times, depicting the scene of an 'overkill'. In the case of Simon, this was clearly evident. The medical reports indicate that his wife had been stabbed seventeen times in the chest and abdominal area. The wounds were severe and the report indicates that the first few blows had lead to her death.

Hyatt-Williams (1996) makes the point that the growing tension or anger within the individual is not always consciously apparent to the offender, or to others, preceding the violent act. Indeed Simon had apparently felt quite resolved about his feelings for his wife at the time of his visit and was sure that they would get back together. By all indications he was excited about the visit and the thought of seeing his daughter.

The affective tension, however, does not simply emerge out of nowhere. It always emerges in response to a perceived threat. As Meloy puts it:

> The mode of violence is clearly affective, delineated by intense autonomic arousal, overwhelming anger during the violence, the perception of the victim as an imminent threat to the ego structure of the perpetrator, a time-limited behavioural sequence and a goal of threat reduction and a return to intrapsychic homeostasis.
>
> (1992, p.47)

Consistent with general observations about rage, mentioned earlier, Meloy makes the point here that the explosive affect mobilized in rage-type murder is ultimately defensive. The aim is to eliminate a perceived threat. In most cases the act is described as a desperate defensive attempt to prevent a disintegration of the personality (Glasser, 1998; Hyatt-Williams, 1998; Meloy, 1992; Menninger *et al.*, 1963; Wertham, 1937). Whether explosive murder is qualitatively or quantitatively distinguishable from other forms of explosive violence still requires further investigation. For instance, it is not yet clear if rage-type murderers, like Simon, experience particular kinds of defences, fantasy or emotion, that set them apart from individuals who are vulnerable to other aggressive reactions or engage in less severe forms of violence. We shall return to some of these concerns later.

A further observation to be made, referring to Meloy's above description, is the use of economic or 'energetic' terminology to describe the affective outburst, thereby referring to it as essentially cathartic in nature. This presumption can be consistently observed across the literature. An unburdening of the tension, as a consequence of the murder, is said to bring great relief to the individual (Meloy, 1988; Revitch and Schlesinger, 1981; Ruotolo, 1968; Wertham, 1937, 1950). Further, symptoms such as dissociation or depression associated with unbearable inner tension tend to remit after the act has been committed. Confessing to the murder, a typical pattern with this kind of murderer, has also been observed to have a cathartic effect (Revitch and Schlesinger, 1981) and perhaps serves as a continuation of the affective discharge after the murder.

It is difficult not to describe explosive violence in cathartic terms as both its objective appearance and the phenomenology of the event point in this direction. But as alluded to earlier, understanding it simply in these terms risks obscuring or foreclosing broader investigation. Although I refer to the use of 'cathartic' terminology in Meloy's work, he is clearly aware of its limitations and emphasizes the role of object relations as well as affective release. Often, however, the significance of the individual's relationship with his surrounding situation and the interactional nature of violence (on an intrapsychic and interpersonal level) are greatly diminished because the act is understood as simplistically based on the cathartic release of aggressive energy. This is reminiscent of Freud and Breuer's (1895) homeostatic drive model where object relationships are not fully accounted for. Simon's case, for instance, makes little sense unless his relationship with his stepmother, its impact (i.e. Freud and Breuer's) on object relations and corresponding affects, and his immediate and enduring situational circumstances are properly understood. The implications of how one contextualizes the affective nature of explosive violence are many. If it were simply a cathartic act, one would expect aggressive eruptions to occur on a regular basis every time the level of aggressive psychic energy peaked. This has implications for treatment and forensic management as one would expect regular repeat offences. However, this does not appear to be the case, suggesting that other factors need to be considered in exploring the matter further. The implications of this line of investigation will be explored further when I consider the intrapsychic features of rage-type murder.

Acute and chronic catathymia

Revitch and Schlesinger (1981) distinguish between acute and chronic catathymia. They divide the explosive act into three phases. Chronic catathymia is most similar to Wertham's original definition where murderous conflict exists within the individual for some time prior to the act itself. This constitutes the first stage of the process, what they have called the *incubation phase*. Here, the individual becomes obsessively preoccupied with his or her victim. The offender-to-be struggles with overwhelming affective states but does not take action. The incubation phase usually lasts several days but can occur for as long as a year. It is usually experienced retrospectively by the individual as a 'dream-like or ego-alien' (p.137) state characterized by inner conflict of both a suicidal and homicidal nature. The second phase, the murderous act itself, is 'triggered by a build-up of tension, a feeling of frustration, depression and helplessness' (p.129) which is then followed by the third phase of the process characterized by a sense of relief.

In acute catathymic homicide, very little time lapses between the eruption of the affective conflict and the act itself. The incubation period is far shorter and may often be a matter of seconds. The internal trigger here is less the build-up of affect, and more simply an experience of sudden overwhelming affect tied to a particular symbolic idea. Revitch and Schlesinger also claim that the third stage differs from chronic catathymia in that the individual usually experiences a flattening of emotions and not a sense of relief. They also contend that in the case of acute catathymia, the victim is more likely to be a stranger and the perpetrator is less likely to retain any memory of the incident. In terms of the type of offender I have worked with, my observations differ slightly from the above. First, although some offenders show signs of inner turmoil when chronic catathymia sets in, there is usually little understanding or acknowledgment of its possible cause. Further, in my experience, their thoughts are seldom of a homicidal nature in terms of a clearly expressed intention to kill. Often, as alluded to earlier, there may be depression or some expression of tension, but there is little awareness of the extent of this inner turmoil. This seems to have been the case in the build-up to Simon's actions.

Second, in terms of acute catathymia, I have not found evidence to support the above claims that such offenders more typically kill strangers and experience greater amnesia. Most of the offenders I have worked with who suffered acute catathymia knew their victims and did not appear to have experienced greater memory loss when compared to chronic catathymic offenders. This, however, is merely anecdotal and I have not measured or tested such claims. Although this is the case it appears likely that these differences could also reflect differences in the type of offender being referred to. My interest in particular offenders who appear 'normal' and do not have a history of violence may explain some of these disparities.

Dissociation

In his attempt to classify different acts of murder, Tanay (1969) uses the term 'dissociative murder' to describe rage-type incidents. For him, the murder is committed in an altered state of consciousness where there is no conscious awareness of the motive for murder. He distinguishes this from two other categories of murder: the psychotic murder and the ego-syntonic murder. The former refers to murders where a florid psychotic episode can be easily observed and where the motive is based on a delusional idea. The ego-syntonic murder, on the other hand, refers to murders with a psychopathic motive where the act does not disrupt the ego functioning of the individual in any way.

Reviewing his earlier work, Wertham (1962) also emphasized the delusional nature of the individual's thinking during the violent act, describing a marked impairment in the individual's contact with reality as part of this process. As

Meloy (1992) suggests, this constitutes a redefinition of the catathymic reaction as a transient psychotic episode where some absence of reality testing can be observed. Meloy argues that this became more apparent to Wertham once an awareness of transient psychotic disorders, evident in such diagnoses as borderline personality disorder, became more prominent in general psychiatric practice. This may well be the case as dissociative experiences of violence associated with borderline phenomena are more readily reported in more recent literature (Hyatt-Williams, 1996; Revitch and Schlesinger, 1981; Gallwey, 1985; Kernberg, 1992).

Further signs that a dissociative process underlies this explosive state are apparent in the offender's description of events following the murder. The individual often lacks insight and is unable to explain, or understand, any motive for the crime. As with Simon, perpetrators often describe their experience of the murder as feeling 'unreal' or 'dream-like'. Another offender, Dan, a successful lawyer who shot and killed his wife and two children after an argument with his wife, had this to say about his actions:

> Its already three years after it [the murder] but I never get emotional about it. I don't really feel things because it still feels like someone else did it. I was in a different state after she shouted at me and something cracked in me, then I was like a robot ... but I could also see myself, as if I was outside of myself, getting the gun and shooting. Apparently I tried to kill myself but I was stopped.

As mentioned in the case of Simon, further signs of dissociation include reports of psychogenic amnesia and the lack of awareness of any lucid violent fantasies towards the individual concerned (Hyatt-Williams and Cordess, 1966; Satten *et al.*, 1960). All this suggests that rage-type murder takes place within an intrapsychic context of dissociation, ego disintegration and depersonalization.

It is often difficult, however, to determine whether the dissociation is part of the cause of the rage-type reaction, or whether it is simply a consequent reaction or way of coping with the ego-dystonic experience that the murder itself represents. This has implications for forensic investigation and legal recourse. Clearly, forensic investigation into the extent to which dissociation occurs is very difficult given that information is always *ex post facto* and eye-witnesses are rare. The extent to which a disturbance in reality testing occurs is also more difficult to assess in these cases given that these kinds of offender are usually compliant, display no odd behaviour and seldom have a history of aggressive behaviour. If one takes the view that the chronicity and level of dissociative experience is proportionate to the level of control and responsibility displayed during the offence, then this becomes an important factor in the legal and psychological management of such cases. In legal terms, it becomes a crucial part of establishing *mens rea* and to what extent *diminished responsibility* is a factor in the murderous act. This is complicated by the fact that sometimes such offenders show few signs of dissociation prior to the crime.

It is often the case that violent offenders claim total amnesia about the incident. This is seldom the case and it is more likely that the offender will recall 'snapshot' images of the events that are experienced as ego-dystonic. This is a useful pattern to look for in individuals who claim diminished responsibility as a result of rage. In my experience, those who claim total memory loss should be regarded with suspicion unless there is clear evidence of psychosis or neurological impairment.

The nature of the dissociative process found in rage-type murder, however, still requires clarification. Dissociation, for instance, has been connected with a number of mental disorders. To what extent, if at all, can these disorders shed light on the type of dissociation observed here? We know that most rage-type murderers are not found to be 'insane' and end up serving normal prison sentences. It has also been established that few rage-type murderers suffer from any form of neurological impairment (Meloy, 1992; Revitch and Schlesinger, 1981; Gilligan, 1996). In other words, the majority of such offenders do not present with attributes which are synonymous with 'insanity' in legal terms. This says little, however, about the possibility of other forms of psychopathology being present in these individuals. We shall consider this problem shortly. In terms of intrapsychic factors, whether these dissociative qualities are chronically entrenched in the personality, part of an acute reaction, or a consequence of the violence itself, will form a substantial part of our investigation of the internal world of such offenders.

Motiveless motivation

Rage-type murder does not appear to have any other motive apart from the explosive expression of aggression that has been triggered by some relatively insignificant event. It is referred to as 'motiveless' not only because there seems to be nothing to be gained by the action, but also because the act appears to be incomprehensible. Stone (1993) takes this to its extreme and suggests that these kinds of murders simply do not have an explanation, and it is this uncertainty in itself that we as health professionals need to tolerate and accept.

In Wertham's initial description of the catathymic crisis, he mentions that prolonged internal tension may lead to a conceived plan to perform a violent act. Wertham is referring here to a more chronic, prolonged rage reaction where a plan has time to be conceived. Less emphasis, however, is placed on this in his later writings (Wertham, 1950, 1962) which appears more consistent with subsequent studies in this area. It is important to note, however, that a plan, or a murderous fantasy, is not the same as a motive for murder. One may become preoccupied with murderous fantasies, and even plan a murder in one's mind, but still not have a motive for carrying it out.

Along with there being no motive, no premeditation is evident and the method of murder is usually described as 'haphazard and impromptu' (Menninger *et al.* 1963, p.239). As is the case with Simon, conventional weapons are often not used in these incidents, an indication of the suddenness of the act. When conventional weapons are used, typically firearms, there is usually no indication that the murder was premeditated.

Revitch and Schlesinger (1981) have put forward perhaps the most detailed account of the specific defining features of different kinds of homicidal act. First, they distinguish the act from neurological and psychiatric conditions, particularly alcohol-induced violence and schizophrenia, which they find only very rarely to be a factor in homicidal behaviour. Then they set out to consider both motivational and dynamic factors in their classification of homicidal behaviour.

Their motivational model places different types of murder on a continuum between endogenous and exogenous motivational factors. They isolate five different types of homicide beginning with the most exogenous type and ending with the most endogenous. It is worth briefly considering these categories.

In the first type of murder, *environmentally stimulated homicide*, exogenous social pressures and controls motivate the individual. Politically motivated murders or murder motivated primarily by social injustices would fall into this category. They are incidental and are less likely to be repeated if the environment changes in some way. In *situational homicide*, Revitch and Schlesinger argue that murder is motivated by a fearful or angry reaction to a stressful situation which may be adaptive. A murder that occurs in an attempt to protect oneself in a threatening situation would be an example of this type. These individuals show few signs of personality disturbance or psychopathology.

In the third type of homicide, *impulsive homicide*, offenders characteristically display very poor impulse control and often have a history of many antisocial acts as a result of this. They differ from situational homicides in that the motivation is primarily derived from a personality predisposition as opposed to being a straightforward reaction to an event. *Catathymic homicide*, the fourth type of murder, is seen as being motivated primarily by emotional outbursts triggered by delusional thinking rather than by any conscious motive. This would exclude murder initiated by some form of obvious or overt threat.

Finally, *compulsive homicide* differs from all the above forms in that such an act is driven by clear fantasy constellations and ideas, predominantly of an infantile sexual nature, that are compulsively acted out. Such individuals have a more coherent personality organization in that violent eruption is less a function of some form of environmental provocation than in other categories of murder.

As Revitch and Schlesinger point out, these are far from discrete categories. In many cases it would be difficult to categorize clearly the act and motivation. Situational murder and catathymic murder, for instance, are difficult to tell apart. They differ, however, in the location of the motivation. Provocation in the situational murder is realistically life-threatening as opposed to the more internal motivation of the catathymic murder. In catathymic or rage-type homicide provocation is minor, or hidden, but serves as a catalyst for other psychological processes that eventually lead to murder.

The endogenous motivations pointed out here have not gone undisputed. Some have argued that the situation under which most explosive murders take place – an argument or a damaging insult – is in itself enough to explain why this kind of murder occurs (Hollin, 1989; Goldstein, 1986). If one argues that the situation essentially accounts for the reaction, then implicit in this suggestion is the assumption that any person in the same situation would react in a similar way. Situational factors thus take precedence over the individual's psychological state. Such a claim largely ignores the complexity of interaction between these two factors.

A study of situational factors and their impact on the individual's psychological make-up bring us closer to understanding the kind of interaction that occurs between external and internal factors. Thus the extent to which we consider this kind of murder to be apparently motiveless is worth exploring further with this interaction in mind. Rage-type murder is mostly considered to be motivated by explosive affect; however, accepting this as the sole motivation does not provide a full explanation for the act and its complexity and, if we are to carry this investigation further, we need other ways of understanding motivation, its source and development. In the previous chapter I have emphasized that violence has multiple dimensions and motivations, all differing in importance depending on the type of violence. It remains to be seen how such dimensions account for rage-type murder.

Situational factors

Turning now to particular situational factors, there appear to be a number of occurrences that regularly emerge. As just mentioned, the interaction between relatively insignificant triggers and the offender's internal world needs to be understood with some caution. External situational factors have an important bearing on what occurs at an intrapsychic level. They are important not only in determining what precipitates the psychological state that ends in murder but also serve as a starting point for understanding what intrapsychic dynamics may have partly created or precipitated the tragic external situation. In other words, the situation not only acts as a determinant, but *why* and *how* such a situation develops may reflect something about the individual's psychological make-up. For example, the availability of a weapon, the number of other people present, or the location may be understood as key determinants as to whether a murder will take place. These same factors, however, may also say something about the perpetrator's intrapsychic life. Why, for instance, was a gun available to Dan? Why did he 'need' to kill his two young daughters who were in no way involved in the incident that precipitated his outburst? To return to the case of Simon, one would also wonder about the unconscious psychological implications of returning to his house and his re-creation of the 'old-times' dinner.

The features emerging from a situational analysis of rage-type murder and its psychological implications would generally be less conspicuous than those of psychopathic or perverse kinds of murder. Perverse murderers act out fantasies and thoughts in a coherent way, etching a clear pattern onto the surroundings and creating a situation from which one can infer much about their psychological make-up. In explosive murder, on the other hand, where there is no motive and it is impulsive, the clues to the individual's internal world become more difficult to discern from the crime scene. The implications this has in understanding the intrapsychic state of the offender will be considered further in exploring the intrapsychic dimensions of violence.

The main situational features often reported in cases of rage-type murder are as follows. Some have already been mentioned in passing.

Innocuous provocation

The offender is typically provoked by a relatively innocuous external event or person that then triggers an acute internal crisis in the offender. Gilligan (1996) argues that the murderous response triggered by such minor provocation is prompted by an acute sense of shame both as a result of the provocation and because the offender feels ashamed of such a strong reaction to a minor incident. As we see with Simon, shame clearly plays a role here. But other factors which we shall explore later, such as the collapse of narcissistic defences and an impoverished representational capacity, are also needed to understand this acute sensitivity.

From an interactional perspective, some have argued that through provocation, the victim contributes to, or has a part to play in, his or her own murder. Abrahamsen (1973), for instance, during the time when a comprehensive body of literature about victims was beginning to emerge, argues that 'the murdered person often plays an unconscious part in his own death' (p.3). As with most of the debate around theories of victimology, this approach is often criticized as an exercise in blaming the victim. This need not be the case; it rather serves as a way of considering the influence of interaction between victim and offender on the violent outcome.

Emotional tie

The offender usually has a close emotional relationship with the victim. In a pioneering study of 588 homicide offenders, Wolfgang (1958) found that over half his sample knew their victims well. As alluded to earlier, this has often been found to be the case in rage offences (Blackburn, 1993; Bowden, 1990; Hollin, 1989; Meloy, 1992). Some researchers, however, notably Menninger et al. (1963) and Stone (1993), report a number of cases where the victims did not know the perpetrator in any way. This appears to be the exception rather than the rule. It is also possible that these cases would be better described as 'psychotic murders' where all contact with reality is lost.

Absence of predation

Predation, or stalking of the victim seldom occurs in rage-type killings. This situational factor becomes important in considering whether there was any form of premeditation related to carrying out an act of murder. It is also an important factor in establishing, more generally, the state of mind of the individual. The individual may, for instance, be plagued by obsessive thoughts about a person leading to predation or stalking. This generally does not occur in rage-type murder. Perhaps part of the reason for this is simply that most explosive murders occur between individuals who have an established, close relationship and therefore predation becomes less of a factor. Given the nature of the relationship, it may also be less reported or a less obvious factor prior to the murder.

Escalating situation

In rage attacks the external situation, and consequently the intrapsychic situation, becomes overwhelming and there appears to be no means of distancing oneself from the interaction. Meloy (1992) describes it as an overwhelming escalation where 'something has to snap'. This again raises important questions pertaining to how such a situation comes about. Does the situation simply occur by chance, or is it co-created in a way that makes it so entrapping? We are all, in some way, over-whelmed by certain difficult situations. It does not follow, however, that we would all commit murder in the same situation. A fraught, provocative or entrapping situation may make us angry, we may even feel 'murderous', but how does this differ from actually carrying out an act of violence or murder?

Overkill

In rage attacks the victim is usually stabbed or shot numerous times, even after the individual has clearly been killed. The 'overkill' nature of the offence has been discussed earlier in terms of the individual suddenly being overwhelmed by explosive affect. Such crime-scene observations may, however, further signify a desperate need in the offender to obliterate either a particular internalized object relationship, or the reality of the situation as it stood at that particular moment. Such action implies a complex set of intrapsychic processes that ultimately lead to murder.

Alcohol

It is often held that the offender was reported to have been under the influence of alcohol at the time of the murder. This is not always a consistent finding. Bowden (1990), for instance, in his review of homicidal behaviour, reports that motiveless murders are rare among alcohol abusers. It is also problematic to view this as a cause for violence as there is no clear relationship to be found between alcohol and violence (Brain, 1986; Collins, 1989; Pernanen, 1991). Given this, alcohol is best understood as functioning like a disinhibitor, making manifest what otherwise may have been controlled. Therefore its role needs to be considered within the context of other variables such as personality (Blackburn, 1993; Pihl and Peterson,

1993). Alcohol may ironically also be used as an attempt to deal with unbearable feelings of rage.

Behaviour after the crime

Often offenders hand themselves over to the authorities after the murder. The situation following the murder is such that the individual is usually shocked and traumatized by what he or she has done but is cognizant of the extreme nature of the situation and thus hands him- or herself over to the authorities. This may be a useful indicator of there being little evidence of psychopathy present in the individual. It should not, however, necessarily be taken as a sign of remorse. The ability to be remorseful or to mourn usually does not occur immediately and only emerges gradually with insight. It also appears that although there is an awareness of the wrongfulness of the act, the relief that occurs after the act serves an important function in preventing the mourning process from beginning immediately. In this sense, relief, if experienced, is not simply about the release of unbearable affect. It reflects a temporary internal state set up by the fantasy that the offender's actions have led to the evacuation and destruction of shameful 'bad' parts of the self. These attempts at disowning parts of the self, to which we shall return shortly, make mourning an impossible process.

CONCLUDING REMARKS

I have outlined the key features that define rage-type murder and raised some of the dilemmas and problems that we face in further understanding this kind of violence. The complexity of the act, however, cannot simply be ascribed to overwhelming destructive affect, dissociative episodes or particular situational factors. These factors are meaningless unless they are viewed within the context of the individual's personality and general life experience. Wertham cogently states this in *A Sign for Cain* where he argues that we cannot separate murderous impulses from murderous people and their context:

> Given the negative emotions, the death wish and the catalyst, there must still be one important factor: the whole personality and the whole life situation of the individual. The difference between one who murders and one who does not is never a simple impulse or a single mental attitude, however destructive.
> (Wertham, 1962, p.40)

Put another way, one might say that the sudden and impulsive nature of the act hides below its surface a complex and timeous preparation. In line with this, the following chapter sets out to consider how mental illness, personality disorders and personal attributes may contribute to the offender's actions.

Chapter 4

Explosive violence, mental illness and personality

> How can a person, as sane as this man seems to be, commit an act as crazy as the one he was convicted of ?
>
> (Satten *et al.*, 1960, p.48)

It is widely accepted that no single personality type or psychiatric disorder can be isolated as being solely responsible for the act of murder. The above statement highlights one of the more perplexing problems we face in understanding the psychology of the rage-type murderer. Often rage-type offenders are described as being apparently 'normal', leaving us with difficulties in understanding why they would commit such a crime. Later, I shall argue that this can largely be attributed to a particular kind of defensive organization used by such offenders.

More generally, however, certain psychological factors do appear related to different types of murder. In this chapter, using both actuarial and clinical findings, I shall explore the relationship between mental illness and explosive forms of violence and then go on to review some of the prevalent personal attributes and personality characteristics that are commonly associated with rage-type murder.

RALPH

Ralph, a 33-year-old man, shot and killed his ex-girlfriend and a friend whilst they sat together in her flat. He walked in, felt them to be a severe threat to him and opened fire until his gun was empty. Three months prior to this, his brother, a security guard, had been killed whilst on duty.

Ralph grew up in a rural village. He was the youngest son of a family of five. His father was a farmer and his mother a housewife. Ralph shared a very close relationship with his mother. He was described, in case reports, as an 'ideal child' who did everything right for his mother and was known for his politeness and good behaviour. Ralph felt that he was very like his mother and often was aware of her presence. He believed that he could see how much they looked alike and claimed that they shared similar gestures. More particularly, he felt he had 'copied' his mother's ways 'in showing people how to be strong and how to help others'.

Ralph felt that he never really knew his father as he was always out working. His father had died when Ralph was 13 years old and from that early age he occupied the position as 'head of the family', took on a lot of responsibility and felt he had to look after his mother. During his schooling years he spent much of his extra time working for money to support her.

His mother died when he was 21 years of age. Following this loss, he still occupied an authoritative position in his family, with family members often turning to him for help. He spent a large amount of his time helping members of his community and doing volunteer work through his local church. A close family friend described his impressions of Ralph as a young adult as follows:

> [Ralph] was often with his mother helping out, he didn't spend much time with other kids, he was, in a way, too old for them and seemed more comfortable with adults. He was always seen by adults as being the 'good kid'. I also remember him being involved in church activities and became particularly active in helping the poorer part of his community.

Ralph's life changed when he won a scholarship to go and study further. During his student career he soon established himself as a well-known student negotiator, dealing with student and staff affairs. He was well known to the head of the institution for his good work in solving problems on campus. One of these cases involved implicating a number of staff members in fraudulent activity. During this period he felt threatened by the conflict that this had caused. He decided to acquired a gun 'just as a precaution and as a means of defence' if he felt 'cornered or in a desperate situation'.

His girlfriend at the time had been a family friend who came from the same village as he did. Ralph had made it possible for her to study through raising funds for her and supporting her at the same college. After 2 years he ended their relationship because she had been unfaithful to him. They parted 'on good terms' with her still doing some of his domestic chores. They maintained regular contact with one another for this reason. After the separation Ralph reported feeling somewhat depressed and wanted their relationship to continue but could not discuss this with her. He felt that perhaps he had done something wrong and he found it difficult not to think about her. On two occasions he felt 'so desperate' that he found himself travelling towards her apartment late at night. On both occasions he turned back before reaching his destination. These shows of distress appeared to last about 2 weeks. After these initial difficulties, however, he was able to resume normal activities, carried on with his studies and never needed to address the feelings he had about his relationship again.

Approximately 6 months later he received a message that his brother had been killed whilst on duty. Ralph was considerably upset by the news but chose not to speak about it to others. In this way, he reported, he 'began to feel much better'.

Three months following his brother's murder, Ralph was invited to his ex-girlfriend's flat to talk about what had happened as she had only recently heard the news. On entering the flat he was asked a 'difficult' question about his brother. Following this he described suddenly feeling threatened by the presence of his ex-girlfriend and another friend who was visiting at the time. He immediately opened fire killing both of them after firing several shots. Once he had arrived, he recalled feeling restless and angry with her for reasons that he could not understand:

> I recall getting to the bottom of the stairs to her flat and I was somehow feeling anger towards her. I had not seen her for sometime, so it didn't make sense. I didn't think about it then though, it was like a kind of deep irritation. But I couldn't think about it because I suppose I had other things on my mind.

Ralph attempted to commit suicide after the act. Prior to this incident no history of violence was reported. Apart from feeling 'depressed' for a short while after his relationship had ended, as well as feeling some anxiety about working as a student negotiator, no other symptoms are evident in his history. He denied having any conscious aggressive fantasies towards his girlfriend.

The prison authorities reported that he was a 'model prisoner'. Shortly after being imprisoned he became one of the main negotiators between the wardens and prisoners.

MENTALLY ILL OR DISORDERED?

How should we understand the above case in terms of mental illness or psychopathology? Was Ralph depressed or psychotic at the time? Did he have a past history of psychiatric illness, something that could have alerted us to the fact that he was capable of committing such a crime? Certainly, although not fully acknowledged by himself, there are a number of stressors apparent in this case that, in part, indicate that he must have been feeling considerably vulnerable at the time of the double murder. But this in itself does not explain why he reacted with such extreme violence.

In cases like this, where there are no obvious motives, there is a greater need to think of the offender as insane. Often such an assumption serves as a means of having some control over the unknown, a way of denying that the offender may have lived an essentially 'normal' life. This kind of reasoning often occurs when murderers are brought to trial and a psychiatric diagnosis is used to mask what is inexplicable. In Ralph's case, for instance, it is tempting to conclude that his brother's death may have induced some kind of pathological state that led to the aberrant attack. But there is little evidence to support this. Certainly he reports being upset, but there is no evidence that this amounted to some kind of diagnosable psychological disorder. Nor did he have a history of psychiatric illness.

Difficulties with the term 'mental illness' have often been pointed out. I shall not discuss these in any depth here (see Kleinman, 1987; McKellar, 1989; Parker *et al.*, 1995). Suffice to say that the inconsistent use of diagnostic categories and the use of non-generalizable samples in diagnostic studies make findings regarding the presence of mental illness difficult to evaluate. For this reason findings in this area should be treated tentatively. These difficulties notwithstanding, to what extent might psychiatric notions of mental illness play a role in understanding rage-type murder, or violence in general? Is there a particular relationship to be found between violent crime and mental illness?

Hollin's (1989) review of research findings suggests that approximately 30 per cent of prisoners have psychiatric disorders. This differs from the general population where an incidence rate of 14 per cent was noted. To contextualize this further, a majority of prisoners are diagnosed with either antisocial personality disorder or a substance abuse disorder (Blackburn, 1993). Specifically relating to homicide, Coid (1983) found the incidence rates of 'mentally abnormal' offenders to be consistent across fifteen research studies. The incidence rates of 'normal' violent offenders, however, varied greatly depending on the socio-political situation in the particular country concerned. This suggests that mental illness can be consistently linked to a particular group of violent offenders. It is important to note, however, that in all the studies reviewed here 'mentally abnormal' offenders only made up a small minority of the cases involved in homicidal acts. This has been supported in a number of other studies (Bowden, 1990; Campbell, 1995; Coid, 1983; Howells, 1982; Howells and Hollin, 1992; Monahan, 1992, 1993; Satten *et al.*, 1960).

Bromberg (1961), in an important early study, claims that most homicide offenders do not show signs of mental illness. He uses the term 'normal murderer', describing such individuals as occasional offenders who had committed a crime 'in response to a solitary aberrant impulse' (p.24). In his words:

> These offenders, not neurotic in the clinical sense, are usually well adjusted, successful persons, without nervous complaints, usually law-abiding, even 'pillars of society,' who inexplicably are propelled into a major crime.
>
> (Bromberg, 1961, p.24)

Certainly, Ralph appears to fit the above profile, often being described as an exceptional student who was highly motivated to help others.

Stone (1993) argues that most offenders, as was the case with Simon and Ralph, are merely referred to a psychiatrist because it is assumed that some 'illness' must be responsible for such heinous acts. He too finds that most murderers do not easily fit into medical classifications of mental illness. A number of other authors have expressed similar observations regarding the apparent normality of these offenders (Goldstein, 1986; Hyatt-Williams, 1998; Satten *et al.*, 1960).

This does not mean, however, that these individuals do not show signs of intrapsychic conflict. Ralph, for instance, displayed a deep investment in an idealized 'negotiator role' that, in later interviews, appeared ostensibly to protect him from dealing with 'dangerous or threatening activities' in his own life. Once this 'benevolent', concerned part of himself was threatened, however, he would become markedly distressed. But to an outside observer, all that was evident was the profile of a helpful, concerned and even righteous individual: to some, the mark of an untroubled 'normal' person. Indeed, Ralph's tragic circumstances left an entire community fumbling for explanations as to why such a model student would commit such a crime.

Two possibilities emerge regarding the apparent absence of psychiatric illness in this kind of offender. First, one might simply conclude that a majority of these individuals are in fact 'normal'. Second, one could argue that this says more about the inadequacies of the present psychiatric diagnostic system in understanding murder. With regard to the latter, I would agree with Revitch and Schlesinger's (1978) statement on the issue:

> Except for the offenses stimulated by paranoid delusions and hallucinations and for the very rare acts of violence committed in states of confusion due to organic or toxic factors and ictal and postictal epileptic states, the psychiatric diagnosis does not explain the offence.
>
> (Revitch and Schlesinger, 1978, pp.138–9)

So far, I have argued that psychiatric illness is not often clearly evident in rage-type offenders and thus cannot account for their actions. Having said that, and although a clinical disorder is not evident in the majority of cases, there is some evidence that suggests that rage offenders have a slightly greater incidence of psychiatric illness. To evaluate these findings further I shall consider some of the main disorders that have been associated with explosive forms of violence.

Depression

Some of the emerging research in this area suggests that there is a link between homicidal behaviour and depression that has been largely overlooked (Blackburn, 1993; Bluglass, 1990; Revitch and Schlesinger, 1981; Rosenbaum, 1990; Rosenbaum and Bennet, 1986).

Revitch and Schlesinger (1981) note that depressive symptomatology is particularly common during the incubation period of the catathymic crisis. Rosenbaum (1990) observes that the depression linked to explosive murder is usually due to a narcissistic injury, in other words, a situation that humiliated or shamed the individual. He contrasts this with an anaclitic type of depression that emerges as a consequence of object loss and the threat of separation. Although this seems consistent with the precipitant factors that produce a rage-type reaction, the distinction between narcissistic depression and anaclitic depression is problematic and difficult to make. This is so because narcissistic injury, triggered by infidelity in Rosenbaum's study, also represents a form of loss related to the self and vice versa. Perhaps it is more useful to conceptualize this relationship on a continuum where the loss of the self is more likely to produce a rage response as opposed to the loss of the object; the former being the more developmentally primitive reaction.

In support of this being a developmentally primitive reaction, Rosenbaum also found that depression was more likely to translate into explosive murder if the individual showed signs of having a personality disorder. Unfortunately he does not specify the type he is referring to. He argues that depressive features are caused by aggressive impulses defensively turned inward which erupt when a trigger event ruptures this defensive strategy. This goes some way in offering an understanding of why explosive offenders are often close to suicide as a result of aggression turned in on the self. It also illustrates how important controlling this defensive strategy becomes to avoid aggressive outbursts.

To return to Ralph's case, although 'depressed' after his relationship break-up, it appears to disappear quickly and there is no clear sign of symptomatology that warrants a full diagnosis. This is often typical of how explosive offenders experience distress or allow it to manifest as we have also seen in the case of Simon. I think that part of the reason for this lies in a number of controlling strategies, including aggression turned inwards, that are typical of the rage offender's personality. We shall return to this idea later in exploring some of the personality characteristics that appear common to such offenders.

Observations regarding depression, however, are not consistent across the research. For instance, in an earlier study, Rosenbaum and Bennet (1986) compared incidents of murder–suicide and homicide and found that although in murder–suicide incidents signs of depression were evident, homicide offenders did not appear to be depressed.

In response to this inconsistency, Collins and Bailey (1990) argue that a more detailed analysis of the relationship between mood disorders and different forms of violence is required. Working with a large prison sample of 1,140 adult males, they found a significant link only between long-standing depression and robbery-related incidents, which they conceptualize as a form of violence. They did not find expressive forms of violence, such as rage-type murder, to be significantly linked to depression. If anything, expressive violence appeared more related to mania than depression.

In order to contextualize these findings further it is important to remember that it is generally accepted that most depressed individuals are passive and non-violent. Further, depression is much more readily associated with suicide than homicide. This suggests that there are a number of other social, interpersonal and psychological factors that need to be considered in these incidents. This is one of the shortcomings of relying on diagnoses as opposed to exploring the more detailed and specific underlying dynamics that are associated with violence.

Psychotic disorders

Hollin (1989), reviewing a number of studies, finds that there is a slightly higher incidence of schizophrenia in offenders who have committed serious offences, particularly those of an extremely violent nature. This has been reported by a number of other authors (Blackburn, 1993; Hafner and Boker, 1982; Howells, 1982; Monahan, 1993; Taylor, 1993). Hafner and Boker (1982) argue that sudden violence may be an important indication of an incipient psychotic process. Further, Blackburn (1993) and Taylor (1993) find that these forms of violence appear to be over-represented in the paranoid group of schizophrenia, but under-represented in the psychoses related to mood disorders. This appears to suggest that violence is more closely associated with the paranoid delusional aspect of psychotic experience, which Taylor (1993) refers to as the 'delusional drive' (p.80) to commit violence.

More specifically, referring to rage-type murder, some have reported a relatively high incidence of psychosis in such offenders. Campion *et al.* (1985), for instance, found that in cases they examined of men who had committed matricide, most of the offenders were schizophrenic. Weiss *et al.* (1960) found that four of the thirteen cases of rage murder they explored showed classical signs of schizophrenia. The other individuals revealed signs ranging from emotional coldness to 'primary process' thinking leading to the conclusion that they too showed signs of psychotic experience. However, the statistical findings are far from consistent and reports related specifically to rage-type murder are lacking. For instance, Taylor (1993), who interviewed 203 violent criminals, found that psychotic individuals were far less likely to engage in extreme forms of violence and were more likely to direct their violent behaviour towards property or non-human objects. She found that most individuals who had been involved in serious crimes, such as murder, did not suffer from a psychotic illness.

As discussed earlier, the act of rage murder often involves transient dissociative or psychotic symptomatology. Ralph reported suddenly feeling both threatened by and angry with his ex-girlfriend but remained baffled as to why he would feel that way. In his words:

> I don't know what happened. I was fine in the car on the way over ... then once I was there I all of a sudden hated her and thought she was going to do something to me. And then I didn't really know where I was or what I had done. The only answer I have is that I must have been possessed by something at the time.

It would be tempting from this to conclude that Ralph's sudden 'paranoia' and disorientation means that Ralph suffered a brief psychotic disorder at the time of the murder. This is especially the case given that psychosis is most readily associated with violence by the media and by the general public (Angermeyer and Matschinger, 1996). There is, however, an important difference between a psychotic murder and a rage-type murder. A psychotic murder is motivated primarily by a battery of paranoid delusional beliefs that preoccupy the individual and precipitate the 'motive' to kill. Rage-type murder, on the other hand, has no apparent motive, delusional or otherwise, and appears to be more directly linked to explosive affect. There also appear to be other differences. Psychotic assaults are often completely unprovoked and may involve bizarre ritualized behaviours (Hollin, 1989; Sohn, 1995; Taylor, 1993). This kind of offender is also more likely to kill a close family member towards whom he or she feels indifferent (Bowden, 1990; Taylor, 1993).

These differences are not often acknowledged in the literature, leaving a confusing picture and making it difficult to understand the relationship between psychotic illness, such as schizophrenia, and rage-type murder. In my view, transient dissociative experiences in the rage offender are better understood as being linked to traumatic experience or as part of the dynamics of the borderline personality. We shall return to this shortly.

Intellectual functioning

Hafner and Boker (1982), in their survey of 533 cases of murder, attempted murder and manslaughter, compared a 'normal' group of offenders with those who showed different forms of psychiatric illness. They found that mentally retarded individuals had more in common with the 'normal' group of offenders in terms of general characteristics. They were also more likely to have experienced a history of family disturbance suggesting that mental retardation itself was not the cause of the violence.

There seem to be two basic relationships between types of offence and intellectual functioning. First, there appears to be a relationship between slightly subnormal IQs and delinquent or antisocial behaviour (Hollin, 1989). Second, individuals who have extremely low IQs display a higher incidence of minor sexual crimes (Blackburn, 1993; Hinton, 1983; Hollin, 1989). However, individuals with subnormal IQs do not appear to have a significantly greater propensity to commit extreme forms of violence such as murder.

Factors related to poor intelligence, such as poor communicative ability, have been found to be important for understanding some forms of violent behaviour. Dura (1997) for instance, found that mentally retarded individuals with poor expressive communicative abilities were more likely to communicate through minor shows of violent behaviour. This probability was found to be greater if associated with some form of frustration and inarticulateness. However, intellectual ability does not appear to be a major factor in extreme forms of violence.

Post-traumatic Stress Disorder

The irritability, fear and hypervigilance which, by definition, accompany the diagnosis of Post-traumatic Stress Disorder (PTSD) may lead to explosive and disruptive behaviour. Solursh (1989), in a study of 100 war veterans suffering from PTSD, reports explosive aggression to be present in 97 per cent of his sample. Collins and Bailey (1990), in a sample of 1,140 prisoners, found that those suffering from PTSD, or symptoms associated with the disorder, were more likely to commit explosive forms of violence.

There appears to be a growing body of research emphasizing the link between impulsive violence and trauma. The idea that violent or murderous behaviour emanates from an original trauma may also be associated with the effects of post-trauma experience, although the individual may not necessarily show signs of PTSD *per se*. Certainly, analysts and psychotherapists, working with individual cases where trauma is evident, have often pointed to the different psychodynamic connections between trauma and aggression or violence. Although Ralph was not directly exposed to trauma and did not report PTSD symptomatology, it is possible that the trauma of losing his brother could have had a significant impact on his mental functioning, making him more defenceless and vulnerable.

In sum then, some psychological disorders, most notably depression and PTSD, appear to endow an individual with a greater propensity for explosive violence. However, this still does not account for the majority of violent offenders who show few signs of overt symptomatology that would suggest the presence of full-blown psychiatric disturbance. Furthermore, although a link between 'mental disorder' and the offence has been supported by some, this does not necessarily mean that a causal link between the two factors exists. As Hollin (1989) points out in his review of earlier research, there are a number of other possibilities: mentally ill offenders are more detectable and thus more readily caught; mentally ill individuals are more likely to be charged; guilty pleas are more readily made by these individuals to ensure treatment. Finally, it is often not clear whether the mental illness is a cause, or whether it occurs subsequent to the offence. For instance, offenders may show signs of PTSD or major depression. However, given the stresses associated with the murder itself, arrest, trial and imprisonment, it is difficult to establish whether these symptoms are a cause or consequence of the offence.

The fact that many of these individuals do not shows signs of having a clinical disorder, particularly psychotic illness, brings us back to the idea of the 'normal murderer'. On the one hand, this brings us face to face again with the idea that anyone, you or I, could be driven to such a sudden extreme. On the other, it leaves us with a number of still unanswered questions specifically related to what 'normal' actually means here. All we have established thus far is that it means that an overt clinical disorder is usually absent. Exploring the personalities and personal attributes of these individuals goes some way in explaining this further.

PERSONAL ATTRIBUTES AND PERSONALITY

There is no single profile that clearly defines the behaviour and personality of the rage-type murderer. Nevertheless, there are a number of characteristics that are common to most.

The first defining personality characteristic occurs by way of exclusion: individuals who have committed rage-type murders do not fit the personality profile of the psychopathic or antisocial personality, a personality type most often associated with violence. Individuals in this category lack the ability to empathize with others, and display a particular form of object relatedness characterized by a perverse form of 'empathy' where emotional connectedness with the external object is maintained through sadistic means. Unlike the psychopath, rage-type murderers seldom have a criminal history, show few signs of sadistic or perverse motives in violence perpetrated, and are not belligerent or impulsive in their general approach.

Satten *et al.* (1960) describe sudden murderers as seemingly 'rational, coherent and controlled, and yet whose homicidal acts have a bizarre, apparently senseless quality' (p.48). The fact that these murders are often described as being out of character also suggests that dissociated split-off aspects of the personality play a part in overwhelming the individual's usual ego functioning. More generally, rage-type murderers have been described as being overcontrolling, rigid and inflexible whilst at the same time prone to sudden disintegration (Hyatt-Williams, 1998; Meloy, 1992; Satten *et al.*, 1960). Their tolerance of any form of affect, particularly anger, is extremely limited lest they be overwhelmed by it. This may explain why, as a means of controlling affect, individuals who have committed rage-type murder often have great difficulty expressing their emotions (Abrahamsen, 1973; Satten *et al.*, 1960). Their relationships with others are often shallow and cold as a result.

This was clearly the case with Ralph. Although a skilled negotiator, he had great difficulty talking about his own feelings and claimed that he could not recall a time that he had become angry. Ironically, although he prided himself in his negotiating skills, he often appeared to use them as a means of controlling his relationships with others in a way that served to avoid potentially conflictual situations. As a result, he would often end up appeasing the other party and was over-compliant in going along with the other person's needs. Simon, in the first chapter, appears to use a similar controlling strategy with his wife by immediately 'forgiving' his wife without dealing with his anger at all. He once said to me:

> I'm not sure I know what anger is. I don't get angry ... See, in my life I have never hated anyone. I always tell myself that if there is any anger between people then you will suffer something terrible. I suppose that's why I seem to want to please others all the time.

Thus anger, or other aggressive emotions, are not usually experienced on a regular basis at a conscious level. Often, such individuals take active steps to avoid aggressive outbursts and are usually very conforming in their behaviour. This does not mean, however, that they are free of destructive impulses. The potentially destructive nature of their personality is evident in reports of them being self-destructive, more accident prone than most and often close to suicide.

Other key characteristics observed in rage offenders include deep feelings of inadequacy, strong dependency needs, as well as an apparent passivity in their general predisposition (Blackburn, 1993; Hollin, 1989; Megargee, 1966). Consistent with this, Ruotolo (1968) also found them to be constantly preoccupied with a sense of isolation and alienation.

In earlier studies, Duncan *et al.* (1958) and Satten *et al.* (1960) found a history of unrelenting physical violence and emotional deprivation in the cases they examined. Long parental absences and a chaotic family background usually characterized emotional deprivation. Many authors, working from different theoretical perspectives, have also found this to be a key factor evident in the offender's history (e.g. Blackburn, 1993; Hyatt-Williams, 1998; Rosenbaum and Bennet, 1986; Zulueta, 1993, 1997). However, consistent with psychoanalytic observations discussed earlier regarding violence in general, a history of abuse or exposure to trauma is not always reported to be present in rage offenders. Blackman *et al.* (1963), for instance, found that the family life of the rage-type murderer was notably cohesive, overprotective and conformist, with no history of abuse. I shall return to considering the role of trauma in Chapter 9.

Classification of violent offenders

There have been some attempts to classify criminal or violent behaviour in order to determine the kind of personality associated with expressive forms of violence such as rage-type murder. The general distinction between 'normal' and psychopathic murderers has already been discussed.

Yarvis (1972) classified criminal offenders into three basic categories, each expressing different forms of aggression. The first group, the *neurotic character group*, is characterized by oedipal conflicts. Here, impulsive behaviour results from a breakdown or rupture of ego functioning as opposed to a more chronic failure to master impulses. Although violence may occur, threatening and damaging behaviour is rare as most of the unconscious rage is deflected away from parental figures onto criminal activity. The second type, the *narcissistic character group*, shows more oral and anal sadistic tendencies, displaying an excessive need to control objects and an intolerance of frustration. Because of this, such individuals are most susceptible to aggressive outbursts when their controlling nature is challenged. In Yarvis' words: 'The rapidity with which the change takes place may be likened to a thundershower – sudden and violent but dissipating quickly' (p.557). He distinguishes this group from his final group, the *ego-disturbance group*, by claiming that forms of violence amongst the narcissistic character group are often deliberate and somewhat controlled. In this way, individuals in this group show more signs characteristic of psychopathic behaviour where violence remains unmitigated by a mature superego. A primitive, narcissistic and dependent form of relating characterizes the ego-disturbance group. They are generally withdrawn, with an extremely low self-esteem. They are incapable of sublimating drive activity and thus explosive outbursts tend to be uncontrolled and frequent because of constant feelings of chaos and instability. This group, he argues, typically represent serial offenders and recidivists who lack the control to refrain from repeat offences.

Central to Yarvis' distinction between the last two categories is the amount of control evident in the personality. The controlling nature of the narcissistic group appears more characteristic of the attributes present in the rage-type offender. I have found the concept of control to be a key factor in understanding the personality of the rage offender. This, of course, is not a new idea in classifying violent offenders, and I shall shortly review some of these observations. The nature of this control, however, and how it manifests in the personality, still requires further investigation from a psychodynamic point of view. How, for instance, does control function in the personality? What essentially is being controlled, and how does this contribute to extreme violence? We shall return to these thoughts later.

Megargee's (1966) classification of violent offenders has been used extensively in criminological literature and has had a great influence on the way we understand the relationship between control and violence. He distinguishes between *under-controlled* and *overcontrolled* violent offenders. The former are characterized by weak inhibitions and impulsivity. As a result, they are prone to regular violent outbursts. He identifies the antisocial personality as being prototypical in this category. The overcontrolled group, on the other hand, display strong inhibitions and only aggresses when some form of instigation occurs. Although violence is evident far less frequently with these individuals, when they are violent they are extremely violent and homicidal. Consistent with this, Blackburn (1971) and Lang *et al.* (1987) found this to be a common feature in homicide offenders. Lang and colleagues further found that homicidal individuals scored lower on general levels of hostility than did general assaultive offenders. This kind of offender is also far less likely to have a criminal record prior to the murderous outburst.

Overcontrolled individuals are therefore usually non-aggressive. On reviewing the typical features of the rage-type murderer discussed so far, it appears that the overcontrolled category best describes these kinds of offender. In sum, they show a high degree of impulse control, low levels of hostility, are markedly defensive and may show signs of depression and inward-directed hostility. It was apparent from my sessions with Ralph that he had always prided himself in his ability to remain in control and 'responsible' at all times. In his words:

> I always make sure that things are in order so I don't get rattled and so things can be kept straight down the line. Also, I could never be aggressive towards others and I always thought that it's because I am

responsible, everyone always told me I was very responsible. I see it [aggression] in others though, and I think I can help them ... but I'm not sure I know what it feels like to tell someone off. I'd rather keep that away from people.

The net effect of this strategy left Ralph feeling quite lifeless and disengaged from others even though he was clearly sociable and had a large network of friends. The control, or overcontrol, in this case was essentially defensive and served to restrict conflict and spontaneous engagement.

Megargee's model of overcontrol does not, however, 'clarify whether it is anger arousal, its expression, or the lack of aggressive habits which are problematic in overcontrolled individuals' (Blackburn, 1993, p.239). In trying to understand this further, Blackburn (1986) suggests that there is evidence of two types of over-controlled individual: first, the *conforming type* are offenders who generally deny anger as an experience and describe themselves as free of anxiety, sociable and conforming. This, he argues, is closer to Megargee's original category. The second type of overcontrolled offender he terms the *inhibited type*. These individuals describe strong experiences of anger but have great difficulty expressing it in any way. They avoid social interaction, report depressive feelings and have a poor self-image.

Blackburn also suggests two similar categories for the undercontrolled group, the *secondary* and *primary psychopathic* groups, which I shall not explore here. What concerns us is whether this kind of categorization of the overcontrolled group further helps in understanding explosive forms of violence or murder. The research in this area is not conclusive at present. Hollin (1989), for example, concludes that this typology appears to hold for the entire offender population rather than just for violent offenders. Notwithstanding this, he does concede that the depressed-inhibited profile appears to be more evident in violent-offender populations.

On the other hand, Hinton (1983), using a behaviour rating scale – the *Objective Behaviour Rating Scale* – for assessing 'dangerousness' in violent offenders, found that overcontrolling, conforming offenders were more highly correlated with murderousness. These individuals were also found far less likely to be associated with other types of criminal offence such as minor assaults. He found this group to be most different from impulsive, belligerent, expressive criminals more closely associated with antisocial characteristics. As opposed to conforming offenders, antisocial offenders were also more likely to have been involved in many different types of offence and these were usually 'non-murderous' in nature. In referring to the overcontrolling individuals who show signs of 'extreme obedience' (p.98) he concludes:

These would seem to be the types who are more likely to have been the domestic killers in real life – the 'bloody handed' as opposed to the 'bloody minded'! They are also more likely to be classified as 'mad' or 'psychotic' as opposed to 'bad' or 'psychopathic'. A high proportion of these killers may never be discharged from security hospital, yet of those who are let out, a particularly low proportion re-offend. In fact, unlike common criminals in general, those convicted of capital offences show little re-offending.

(Hinton, 1983, p.98).

The point he takes up here about re-offence appears to be reasonably well supported in the literature (Blackburn, 1993; Carney, 1976; Howells and Hollin, 1992; Meloy, 1992; Menninger *et al.*, 1963), although many have noted the complexities and problems related to predicting violence or dangerousness (e.g. Campbell, 1995; Limandri and Sheridan, 1995; Milner and Campbell, 1995; Prins, 1990). As to whether rage-type murderers belong more to the conforming group as opposed to the inhibited group there appears to be no decisive criminological research that clearly places explosive murder in one or the other.

From my own clinical experience I have found the conforming aspects of the personality to be a more prominent feature of how affect and object relationships are controlled by the individual. Here, obedience, conformity and appeasement appear to serve crucial defensive functions aimed at controlling perceived bad or shameful aspects of the self. My understanding of control is slightly different from Megargee's in that it is not only impulses that are controlled or restricted, but also external and internal objects. In other words, impulses cannot be seen in isolation from their aim or object. Furthermore, this view emphasizes the fact that over-control has both interpersonal and intrapsychic consequences. I shall say more about this when we explore the particular defensive strategies used in these cases.

So far we have explored how explosive violence can be explained mainly in terms of criminological typology and personality attributes. I turn now to considering how these features compare, if at all, with the designated personality disorders used in psychological literature.

Personality disorders

Personality disorders, as opposed to symptomatic psychiatric illness, are generally viewed as being a much better predictor of violent behaviour. Broadly, the term 'personality disorder' refers to structural character deficits in the personality that lead to enduring patterns of maladaptive behaviour. In reviewing the literature in this area one of the main difficulties one comes across is the confusion that has occurred in the use of terminology. As a result, and depending on one's theoretical understanding and emphasis on behavioural or psychodynamic characteristics, many different types of personality disorder have been alluded to in discussing explosive forms of violence. Most, however, essentially refer to similar factors, suggesting that it is the confusing use of terminology, rather than there being many different types of personality disorder involved, that is the problem here.

Some authors have simply used the term 'personality disorder' to refer to an unspecified category in acknowledging the influence of structural deficits in the personality when referring to rage-type murderers (Carney, 1976; Revitch and Schlesinger, 1978; Rosenbaum, 1990). Others have implicated particular types of personality disorder. Meloy (1992) argues that psychotic or borderline personality organizations explain most homicidal acts. Likewise, Blackburn (1993) finds that borderline personality disorder is an important consideration in understanding general acts of violence. Apart from antisocial personality disorder, most readily associated with violent behaviour, Kernberg (1984, 1992) associates narcissistic and borderline personality disorders with sudden aggressive behaviour. A number of authors also describe what would more typically be referred to as a schizoid personality disorder (Hinton, 1983; Menninger *et al.*, 1963; Ruotolo, 1968).

An added confusion in referring to personality disorders results from the *Diagnostic and Statistical Manual of Mental Disorders IV*'s (American Psychiatric Association, 1994) categorization based on behavioural and observable criteria. This differs greatly from how such terms were originally used to describe common psychodynamic processes in the personality. Categorizing personality disorders as distinct behavioural entities misses the point in the sense that many of these disorders share similar underlying psychodynamic features. This is highlighted when one attempts to use the *DSM-IV* to understand some of the characteristics of the explosive personality discussed so far. Many different personality disorders appear to be partially implicated, but none stand out as a precise description of the kind of problem evident in the rage-type murderer. This leaves us with no clearer a picture than we started with. For instance, the schizoid, avoidant and dependent personality disorders all tend to allude to the constricted, withdrawn and isolated aspects of the explosive personality, whilst both the borderline and narcissistic personalities best explain the sudden emotional outbursts characteristic of the act of rage-type murder.

Blackburn (1993) tries to address this problem to some extent by proposing a dimensional classification system for personality disorders, bringing together some of the criminological and psychological literature in this area. Here, the over-controlled group is characterized by dependent, compulsive, avoidant, schizoid and passive aggressive personality types. Significantly, Blackburn is unsure where to place borderline personality disorder in his classification attempt. Perhaps this is understandable given the very confused and broad way the term is used. It may equally reflect the difficulties in using this term to describe a constellation of behaviours and symptoms without referring to the underlying psychodynamic features of the personality.

I want to consider borderline personality disorder in more detail here as it appears to be most often implicated in explosive forms of violence. This is especially the case when the underlying structural dynamics of the personality are taken to be the main categorizing factor.

Unfortunately the confusing use of terminology does not disappear when one focuses simply on psychodynamic processes. This is especially the case with the borderline personality. Borderline personality is sometimes used interchangeably with the schizoid personality (Fairbairn, 1952; Rey, 1988) and the narcissistic personality (Bateman, 1998; Rosenfeld, 1971, 1987). In some cases, it is also used to refer to a spectrum of conditions and is not regarded as a single disorder (Kernberg, 1984; Stone, 1980).

I shall not discuss this in any depth here but turn to exploring the use of the term with reference to explosive violence and rage-type murder. A comprehensive overview of the borderline personality can be found elsewhere (Jackson and Tarnopolsky, 1990; Kernberg, 1992; Stone, 1980). For the sake of clarity, Kernberg's (1984) use of the term will be employed here. His flexible, but precise, description of the different dynamic configurations of the borderline personality appears most suited to the characteristics of the rage-type offender discussed thus far.

In Kernberg's view, the borderline personality organization covers a number of different character manifestations that share the same underlying structural dynamics and developmental characteristics. Symptoms are not considered in isolation but point to important structural deficits in the personality apparent in narcissistic, schizoid and antisocial personalities, if one uses the *DSM-IV* classification system. The common structural features relate to a chronic, diffuse identity that is dealt with by using primitive defence mechanisms. Self representations and object representations remain contradictory and have not been integrated into a coherent identity typically found in the neurotic personality.

As a result, borderline individuals fail to obtain real empathy and maintain superficial, chaotic or blocked relationships with others. The defensive system used here involves splitting, projective identification, idealization, denial, omnipotence and devaluation. The many different ways in which the primitive defensive system is used makes the overt appearance of the borderline organization appear so diverse. The identity diffusion which occurs here is not as great as that found in the psychotic personality where boundaries between the object and the self are much more tenuous.

To return to the personality features of the rage-type murderer, there appear to be two common trends in the literature that can be understood in terms of Kernberg's borderline category. The first is found in Satten *et al.*'s (1960) description of the offender as having poor impulse control, transient blurring of fantasy and reality, altered states of consciousness, shallow or blunted affect and, finally, a violent and primitive fantasy life. Meloy (1992) also describes similar erratic and impulsive features in the detailed description of a woman who committed a catathymic murder. He uses the term 'borderline catathymia' to describe the case. These descriptions are most similar to the *DSM-IV*'s diagnosis of borderline personality disorder.

In contrast, the other, perhaps more common description characterizes the individual as having severe deficits in the personality but with a much more controlled outward appearance. The ostensibly 'normal' personality discussed earlier appears to correspond more closely with this description. Certainly, Megargee (1966), Blackburn (1993) and Hollin's (1989) descriptions of the overcontrolled personality seem to suggest this kind of presentation.

The disparity between accounts of the more impulsive, incoherent personality and the overcontrolled version, may simply be a consequence of whether the individual is under any kind stress or not at that point in time. This appears to be the case with Meloy's (1992) description where the offender's history appears to be a lot more stable and controlled prior to the onset of the more incoherent catathymic turmoil. Satten *et al.* (1960) also write about the apparent normality of such individuals despite their being impulsive at times.

In the majority of cases I have worked with, the 'stable' outer shell is markedly evident but is always under threat of sudden collapse if their defensive system is compromised. Notwithstanding this, men like Ralph manage to live relatively stable lives, both in the workplace and at home. Although it is not always a measure of 'stability', some of these men also managed to achieved great success, usually in the workplace or on the sports field. I mention this because in these cases 'success' appears to be motivated by idealization and the need to deny bad conflictual experience. One of Ralph's student colleagues had this to say about his achievements: 'He was always busy, that's why he was successful at anything he tried, he was always over-working, he was a perfectionist. He was always very serious about what he did and never ran out of energy.' Although this is mentioned in a positive light, in terms of Ralph's unwavering abilities, his 'success' here, I believe, also sheds some light on his propensity for explosive violence. Later, I will put forward the idea that a complex system of vigilant defences partly explains this apparent stability.

There have been some attempts to conceptualize the psychodynamics of this apparent stability. Under the broad heading of the borderline personality, Gallwey (1985) discusses two different types of dual personality organization that may exhibit violent or homicidal behaviour. These organizations are similar to Deutsch's (1942) discussion of the 'as-if' personality: what Winnicott (1965) later called the False Self personality. Although they say little about the actual dynamics of violence related to these organizations, the structural features of this personality type appear to explain some of the features of the potentially explosive individual.

Gallwey wishes to emphasize the paradoxical characteristics often associated with the 'borderline' concept where apparently relatively well-adapted individuals exhibit bouts of disturbance not congruent with the rest of their personality. His emphasis on the apparently normal and adaptive nature of the borderline personality resonates with the conforming, overcontrolling and non-revealing attributes of the explosive personality described earlier. Both personality types are shielded by a pseudo-personality that appears relatively adaptive and may at times exhibit neurotic symptomatology. It is this general dynamic that often leaves one surprised when these individuals display disturbed behaviours as it seems incompatible with their apparent normal functioning.

Jackson and Tarnopolsky (1990), in their review of the borderline concept in forensic psychiatry, support the above claim. They have this to say about such offenders:

the most severe, and at times most unexpected, psychopathology relevant to the forensic field is found in a group of 'pseudonormals', who have very severe and encapsulated psychopathology. Although able to function well under normal circumstances, they are prone to outbursts of bizarre and dangerous behaviour when their powerful splitting defenses give way.

(Jackson and Tarnopolsky, 1990, p.432).

They differentiate this type of 'pseudo' personality presentation, characterized by extreme destructiveness, from the majority of borderline individuals who more readily display inadequate and deprived personalities.

CONCLUDING REMARKS

In reviewing psychiatric illnesses that may be associated with rage-type murder, I have argued that psychotic illness is seldom evident in the rage-type murderer. Psychotic dissociative symptoms are transient and appear better explained as a feature of the borderline personality structure. Although poor intellectual functioning may play a role in some crimes, it does not appear to be associated with explosive murder. Depressive and post-traumatic conditions, on the other hand, appear to be more readily associated with rage-type murder, although it is, at present, difficult to understand the temporality of such conditions. Broadly speaking, however, psychiatric illness, as a feature of the offender's psychological make-up, does not appear in the majority of offenders and thus is limited in its explanation of the offence.

In reviewing the personality characteristics of the rage-type offender, I have suggested that certain characteristics appear common to most of these offenders. Most notably they appear ostensibly 'normal'. The research in this area, from criminological and psychological perspectives, suggests that an overcontrolled pattern of behaviour may explain this. Whilst pointing out the difficulties in the definitions of personality disorders, I have attempted to draw some links between this overcontrolled pattern and a specific kind of borderline personality. The idea of a dual personality structure appears to go some way in forming a basic theoretical understanding of the rage offender. However, the quality of the object relations and defences used here, as well as the role of other intrapsychic dimensions, still require further exploration. How we should understand explosive affect related to violence and murder in the context of this 'overcontrolled' personality structure is also not clear. Before considering these questions in close relation to my own work, let us consider how others have understood the psychodynamics of explosive murder.

Chapter 5

Formulations of rage-type murder: past and recent contributions

Throughout the development of this research area authors have broadly agreed that murderous impulses originate from an internally threatened part of the personality that attempts to ward off danger through the annihilation of what is perceived to threaten the individual. The act is clearly affective and self-preservative in nature. Views differ, however, concerning the specific psychodynamic nature of the act, as well as the premorbid intrapsychic qualities evident in the personality.

Beginning with Wertham's catathymic crisis and moving on to more contemporary formulations, I shall isolate key ideas that have been put forward to explain the act. The formulations I have chosen all emphasize different aspects of the problem, in turn leading us closer to further questions that require exploration.

EARLY DEVELOPMENTS

Wertham: the catathymic crisis

We have already discussed some of the clinical and dynamic qualities that Wertham attributed to the act of rage murder. Briefly, he found there to be a marked period of ego-centricity and build-up of affect attached to a particular unresolvable idea which eventually leads to a violent cathartic response. In a later contribution, *A Sign for Cain*, Wertham (1962) warns that it is misleading simply to emphasize the impulsive nature of the killing. His statement, 'Nothing has a longer preparation than an impulsive violent act' (p.42), paves the way for the consideration of other psychological factors that contribute to such an offence.

Wertham makes no distinction between those who commit violence and individuals who commit murder. He argues that hate and consequential fear are key factors that create an oversensitivity in violent individuals. As Wertham puts it, 'Cause fear and you sow the idea of violence' (p.37). In a transient form, this is not an uncommon experience for most of us. Prolonged hate, however, causes even greater sensitivity and murder itself is seen as a fantasized end to these distressing emotions. The point is, however, many of us may think of violence in the face of fear, but, as Wertham concedes, it is much more difficult to understand why some go to the extreme of committing murder.

Two more factors can be isolated in Wertham's work with murderers that may be seen as an attempt to understand this problem further. First, he finds that they possess a particular kind of 'magical' thinking that is 'supremely arrogant. The persons are habitually disposed to lift themselves, not by work or thought but by some quick action against others' (p.35). Underneath this, however, and this brings us to the second factor, he finds that these individuals often feel inferior, incompetent and are extremely passive. Violence or murder, he argues, frees them from these disabling factors in the personality.

Wertham struggles to make any further headway in understanding the intra-psychic qualities of rage-type murder. In concluding, he argues that it is often simply about an 'unsolvable' internal problem which incidentally, via the media or through interaction with others, becomes fused with the 'easy' or 'magical' solution of murder which is then carried out. He acknowledges that such an explanation would be viewed as superficial by most but also cautions about equating the extreme nature of the crime with a greater need for a 'deeper' understanding. Although this is an important point, it does not address the need for further under-standing regarding the predisposing intrapsychic nature of the personality. Instead of further exploring these possibilities, he turns to external factors such as alcohol, poverty and the accessibility of weapons to explain violence. Again, although these are undeniably significant factors, he does not consider their intrapsychic causes or consequences and thus forecloses further exploration in this area.

Menninger and colleagues: episodic dyscontrol

Menninger's understanding of murderous rage grew out of a large body of work, beginning in 1928 (only published in 1973), dealing with different aspects of destructiveness and aggression (Menninger, 1942, 1966, 1973; Menninger and Mayman, 1956; Menninger et al., 1963). In his first case study involving an appar-ently normal individual who kills his wife, Menninger (1973) views murder as a symptom of extreme psychological isolation. According to him, the typical rage-type murderer also has a history of episodic impulsive acts of violence.

Menninger and his colleagues characterize these individuals as having severe ego disturbances not typical of neurotic disorders. At the same time, they found that these individuals did not fit psychotic, borderline or schizophrenic descrip-tions. Menninger identifies two prodromal factors that represent the first two lines of defence before murderous rage erupts. First, neurotic defences are increasingly employed but fail to dissipate anxiety. Second, some evidence of paranoid experience and its accompanying defences begins to occur. The naked display of aggression represents a third line of defence against further disorganization and destruction of the personality. In this way, although aggression is depicted as being uncontrollable, it still performs a crucial function.

Although Menninger's focus is on ego control, he shares similar ideas to those put forward by Wertham regarding the psychodynamics of the act itself. The act is driven by a build-up of affect or psychic energy that has a cathartic or relieving effect after a rupture in the ego has occurred. It amounts to the general assumption that the personality is governed by homeostatic principles first considered by Freud and Breuer (1895) in their discussion of the *constancy principle*. Briefly, this refers to the assumed tendency for the psyche constantly to return to a level of minimal stimulation through the discharge of affects that disrupt the homeostasis. This idea was modified considerably by Freud, but the essence of the principle remains relevant to Menninger's assumptions about explosive rage, or what he calls episodic dyscontrol. The metaphors that Menninger uses: flooding an area to prevent an overfilled dam from overflowing; or the need to incise an abscess to prevent it from getting further infected, convey an understanding of the event that is fundamentally about economic principles. Viewed in this way, the ego and 'pure' affect are constantly being played off against each other with insufficient attention being given to the role of object relations in the build-up to violence and the murder itself.

In emphasizing the structural economic principles behind murderous rage, both Wertham and Menninger implicitly separate affect or 'psychic energy' from under-lying object relations that make up the personality. In doing so, they foreclose further exploration of the specific nature and function of other psychodynamic factors and general personality characteristics. As already pointed out, the fact that explosive violence, especially murder, does not occur on a regular basis in a constant attempt to restore a homeostatic balance in the personality suggests that many other factors, internal and external, require consideration here. They cannot be viewed as secondary to the constancy principle. Although this principle may accurately *describe* reports of how extreme rage is experienced and the relief that follows, the analysis of the event or its prodromal factors cannot be based solely on our conscious experience. A fuller analysis of the underlying factors that contri-bute to this experience is needed.

To be sure, Menninger is clearly aware of the particular psychodynamic make-up of each case he explores. He finds, however, that 'these dynamics do not explain the extremity of the act, the violence and the apparent meaninglessness of the act' (p.239). He argues that these eruptions have a more general economic implication: they function as an attempt to prevent something worse happening within the personality.

In other publications specifically related to sudden murder in which Menninger is a co-author, some psychodynamic factors are outlined. Satten *et al.* (1960) argue that sudden murder is caused by 'severe lapses in ego control which make possible the open expression of primitive violence, born out of previous, and now uncon-scious, traumatic experiences' (p.48). Studying the history of four cases of murder, they conclude that the overwhelming nature of early traumatic events prevents any form of ego-mastery from occurring causing 'early defects in ego formation and severe disturbances in ego control' (p.50). As a result, the ego is left deficient, brittle and inflexible. They also contend that this may, at times, lead to a tendency to over-control elements of the personality. The extent to which this reflects the same kind of overcontrol discussed in the previous chapter remains unclear.

As a consequence of having inflexible ways of managing emotional experience, the overcontrol Satten and his colleagues are referring to here appears to serve as a means of keeping relationships devoid of emotional experience. They describe the relating capacity of such individuals as follows:

> Their relationships with others were of a shallow, cold nature, lending a quality of loneliness and isolation to these men. People were scarcely real to them, in the sense of being warmly and positively (or even angrily) felt about.
>
> (Satten *et al.*, 1960, p.51)

They further found that all the men who were studied displayed a 'bizarre, violent and primitive fantasy life' (p.50) evident mostly in repetitive violent dreams. A distinction is made between this and conscious fantasy, claiming that conscious fantasy and ideational material was minimal in such offenders. Dissociation and depersonalization were also reported by these men, but this was not given any specific dynamic meaning.

In sum then, apart from emphasizing the role of ego dysfunction, the Menninger group also found the role of trauma to be significant in rage murderers. No single unconscious motive could be found for these kinds of killing apart from a general desperate attempt to avoid further disintegration of the personality. In essence, sudden murder occurs when a lapse in ego control allows for the reactivation of an old conflict where the victim becomes a key figure.

Bromberg: 'the cuckolding reaction'

Bromberg (1961) speaks of the murderous incident as a creative experience where 'a criminal act succeeds in organizing, perhaps for a fleeting instant, a new set of life arrangements, new emotional configurations and so on' (p.9). Although the use of the word 'creative' is somewhat problematic given that it is a destructive act, he explains: 'a destructive act is a creative act when viewed from the individual standpoint. It accomplishes aims consonant with the total configuration of his inner drives' (p.10). Again, his views do not differ much from Wertham and Menninger in terms of general structural dynamics; he sees sudden murder as resulting from ego dysfunction and the failure of repression.

In addition, Bromberg found that explosive murders are usually related to an intense unconscious fear of being exposed as sexually inadequate. Offenders, he claims, are constantly preoccupied with ways of defending their own sexual virility and an extremely high emotional charge surrounds this sexual fear. Bromberg calls the psychological mechanism through which this reaction takes place the 'cuckolding reaction' (p.29). The cuckolding sign, made by putting the thumb between the first and second finger, is an ancient symbol of hypersexuality and when thrust at someone represents disdain for sexual impotency or inadequacy. Here, murder is a last-ditch reactive attempt at eliminating the perceived cause of extreme feelings of sexual inadequacy.

Bromberg thus places explosive or rage murder squarely in the realm of the Oedipal Complex. He relates the extreme humiliation that results from the exposure of sexual inadequacy to a repressed homosexuality originally involving the father. For this reason these murders are usually enacted within a triangular situation resulting in two different outcomes. Either the offender destroys his love object for betraying his (unconscious) shared secret about his inadequacy by seeking someone else and leaving the offender exposed. Or, second, the male 'competitor' is attacked in an act of triumphant rivalry. The greater the oedipal insecurity the more violent the reaction

In an earlier paper, however, involving a detailed reconstruction of a case of explosive murder complicated by alcoholism, Bromberg (1951) highlights the role of early oral aggression. In this case, destructive phantasies were more about aggression towards unborn children, fear of a castrating mother, revenge against women, and less about typical oedipal fears. Further, compliance and passivity are seen as a character defence against unconscious aggressive impulses. Bromberg concludes that the murder was a defensive reaction against overwhelming passivity which the offender unconsciously shared with women through identification with them. Therefore, it is the passive feminine object that is annihilated. Here, the core insecurity appears to stem from internal dynamics between the offender, the maternal object and his identification with her.

The precarious nature of identifications certainly appears to add to a chronic, although hidden, sense of insecurity in these individuals. This is evident in both the cases previously discussed. Although both Simon and Ralph give the impression of having a reasonably robust exterior, a closer analysis makes it apparent that they both struggled to establish a stable sense of identity and self-direction. Simon, in particular, spent a great deal of psychic energy rebuking anything that closely resembled an identification with his stepmother. I shall argue later that one of the intrapsychic precipitants of rage emanates from a forced or intrusive identification with internalized bad objects once narcissistic defences have collapsed. The intrusive identification is felt to be particularly devastating due to a poorly established sense of identity resulting from a flight away from establishing stable identifications because the process is inculcated with fear.

Bromberg's study raises important questions regarding the role of the 'cuckolding reaction' in preoedipal object relations. His work reflects the general problems evident in attempting to conceptualize the influence of both oedipal and preoedipal experience in understanding particular behaviours or mental states (Grotstein, 1981; Westen, 1989). I suggested earlier that the level at which these themes are represented in the psyche appears to provide a better indication of how both oedipal and preoedipal factors influence psychic activity.

Weiss and colleagues: the dependency trap

Weiss *et al.* (1960) provide one of the most detailed earlier accounts of the psychodynamic factors evident in the prodromal personality of the sudden murderer.

In a comparative study of 13 habitual offenders, 13 sexual offenders and 13 sudden murderers, they report the following characteristics as being typical of the sudden murderer: their family backgrounds were characterized by a poor relationship between parents but the families remained an ostensibly cohesive unit; fathers were always found to be hostile or indifferent; the mothers occupied a domineering, conforming and overprotective role.

Weiss and colleagues believed that the mother's overprotective behaviour constituted a reaction formation to her own aggressive feelings towards her children. Further, these future murderers found themselves in a situation where they could not adequately identify with a paternal figure because of the father's overt hostility. As a result, they remained strongly attached to, and in partial identification with, the mother's strong dependency needs and her need for conformity. In order to maintain this attachment, and in an attempt to preserve some love, all reactive feelings of hostility towards the mother were repressed. Their internal world is characterized by considerable insecurity. On the one hand, their maternal identification leads to sexual identity problems, on the other hand, they cannot turn away from this for fear of breaking with their mother's conforming ethos and risking losing her love.

As a result, Weiss and colleagues argue that these individuals internalize a strong need to conform and succeed. However, because of their insecurities and confusion regarding their own identity and underlying hostility, they constantly fail. This sets up a cycle of personal failures that leads to escalating feelings of anger and rage. Because they are unable to deal with failure, it is projected in the form of constantly blaming the 'bad world' for their own insecurities.

Interestingly, Weiss and his colleagues also found that rage-type murderers displayed a period of overt healthy adjustment for a duration, ranging from a month to a year, before the murder took place. For instance, the individual may have kept a steady job or relationship for a reasonable length of time. This appears to be significant in that conformity brings with it more pressure to succeed, thus widening the gap between real feelings of inadequacy and the demands of conforming to a task. Further, the individual is no longer armed with defensive manoeuvres that aim to blame others, as he or she is succeeding. In this way they are forced closer to confronting their own unbearable self.

This is the source of the inner turmoil that eventually, when triggered by minor provocation, leads to the sudden murder. The provocation feeds the inadequacy that the individual can no longer tolerate, leading to 'the ultimate projection, a feeling of "I am no good, but it's your fault!"' (p.674). This constitutes an ultimate attempt to rid himself of the bad object that always reminds him of his intolerable inadequacies.

It is important to note, however, that Weiss finds that part of what makes these inadequacies inescapable is the unsuccessful use of projection because these murderers have become too overtly aware of their own deficits. Thus they are unable to keep them at a distance by projecting them into another object. In this sense, the 'ultimate projection' might be seen as a final violent attempt to instil and fix what they desperately want to disown into another person. I would agree with Meloy (1992) in pointing out that projective identification seems better to describe this action, where homicide becomes an ultimate form of control over the devalued victim/projected part of the self. This thinking goes hand in hand with broader developments in psychoanalytic thinking to which we will return in considering some of the more recent contributions in the field.

In a later study by the same research unit, Blackman *et al.* (1963) emphasize intense conforming and dependency needs present in the 43 cases they review. Dependency needs, however, are vigorously denied and explosive bouts of rage become the ultimate means of denying this need. They emphasize this as the key to why the murder takes place: 'The offender is aware of his own dependency needs, but he tries to deny them; the explosive reaction of rage becomes the ultimate brutal denial' (p.293). The façade of independence used to ward off these feelings eventually becomes impossible to uphold.

Ralph and Simon both appear to illustrate the above point. It could be argued that both men had great difficulty acknowledging dangerous dependency needs that surfaced only once they had felt threatened and vulnerable. In addition, however, dependency and conformity appear to play a much more fundamental role in their general defensive strategies. Here, dependence on the object, often disguised as some form of benevolence, forms part of a desperate means of taking flight from their own hazardous internal worlds. We shall explore this later in considering how this forms part of the defensive organization that is typically found in such offenders.

Ruotolo: the damaged pride system

Ruotolo (1968), in 'Dynamics of sudden murder', investigates five cases of sudden murder. With slightly different emphases on the dynamic features described above, he views the murderous response as a reaction to a perceived irrevocable assault on an idealized self-image or 'pride system' (p.173) that desperately needs to be upheld. The assault or blow generates intolerable self-hate which is then externalized onto the victim in a desperate attempt at restoration of the self. In this sense, the preservation of the 'pride system', as opposed to the obliteration of the object, is primary here. In his words, 'Some personalized value was found to take precedence over the "ultimate" crime of murder. The *sine qua non*, this unique image of oneself, had to be maintained by the murderer at any price' (p.162).

Ruotolo's findings appear very similar to the kind of rage that occurs in response to narcissistic injury. The shame and humiliation that results leads to extreme hate and, in Kernberg's terms, a 'radical devaluation' (p.23) of the object leading to murder or suicide. A number of authors have since supported this claim (Frazier, 1974; Gilligan, 1996; Rosenbaum and Bennet, 1986). Rosenbaum and Bennet (1986) for instance, found that homicidal impulses were essentially linked to narcissistic injuries that led to a sudden drop in self-esteem, whereas Frazier (1974) associated explosive murder more with milder, repeated humiliations accompanied by feelings of shame.

To refer back to the case of Simon. He was victim to repeated bouts of humiliation from his stepmother that could be understood in this way. As he grew up he worked very hard to build up a 'pride system' that was ultimately defensive and dangerous if tampered with. As he put it: 'I was proud of myself after I left [his stepmother], proud of what I had done. From then on I was doing good things and no one could touch that. No one dare take that away from me.' But the circumstances that followed did exactly that, prodding an already shamed and damaged part of himself, in turn triggering a repetition of accumulated humiliation and consequential self-hate.

The self-hate that results from narcissistic injury sets the scene for further self-destructive behaviours, a common feature in all of Ruotolo's cases. He also notes what he describes as a 'seeming indifference to their own lives' (p.74). As well as being emotionally isolated from others, he appears to refer here to a sense of these offenders being alienated from their own affective states, especially anger.

Ruotolo outlines a second dynamic component to sudden murder: there is a move away from a neurotic solution, in which symptoms are used to play out particular conflicts, to a repressed solution characterized by self-effacement. Repression, however, cannot be maintained and causes extreme anxiety that, in turn, precipitates a desperate need to return to a neurotic solution. The potential for murder occurs when the victim unknowingly stands in the way of the offender returning to his previous mental state. However, Ruotolo is somewhat sceptical about his own assumptions here as first, a number of these cases did show evidence of secure neurotic solutions and second, four of his cases presented with fragile ego boundaries and signs of psychotic breakdown. As Meloy (1992) suggests in his review of this study, the above characteristics appear to resemble closely the dynamics of a borderline personality organization.

In sum then, the murderous act occurs not so much because the victim happens to 'fit' into preconceived object relations, phantasies and unconscious conflicts that are re-enacted. It is more a reaction than a re-enactment. Murder occurs because victims are felt to be symbolic impediments to the restoration of 'pride' and a more tolerable psychic state. According to this view, the victim is seen one-dimensionally as an obstacle to recovery. The significance of the object's particular characteristics for the offender's internal world are not seen as an important dynamic feature of this kind of murder. This view differs somewhat from the main view that some form of transference enactment takes place when these murders are committed (Hyatt-Williams, 1998; Meloy, 1992; Revitch and Schlesinger, 1981).

RECENT CONTRIBUTIONS

The above approaches differ considerably in emphasis. However, a number of themes emerge from these earlier studies. Notably, their formulations are mostly based on the idea of homeostasis where murder is propelled by aberrant affect that, in turn, serves to restore a psychic balance. The above formulations also consistently describe the offender as being dependent, compliant, passive and extremely insecure. On the other hand, in an almost contradictory way, the offender is also viewed as being 'independent' and somewhat arrogant in disposition, depicting a more 'stable' but removed self. The later formulation, however, perhaps with the exception of Weiss *et al.* (1960), is not clearly developed and no consolidated attempt is made to build the 'apparent normality' of the offender into their understandings. The personality profile of the offender is also not clearly developed.

Although in more recent studies the homeostatic model does not disappear altogether, more emphasis is placed on the role of internal objects, their corresponding affective valences, and more primitive psychological processes such as splitting and projective identification. There is some agreement here that borderline personality organization best describes the intrapsychic processes involved. I suggested earlier that a particular type of borderline personality appears to typify best the 'overcontrolled' nature of the offender. Whilst this is implicit in some of this work, it still remains under-formulated along with the 'apparent normality' and general profile of the offender. I shall explore some of the key elements of these formulations before taking the investigation further. I consider Reid Meloy and Arthur Hyatt-Williams to be pioneers in this area and confine myself to their contributions.

Meloy: pathological attachments and borderline personality organization

Following Revitch and Schlesinger (1978), Meloy develops a broader understanding of the psychodynamics of catathymic murder by using attachment theory combined with an object-relations perspective. Drawing on more recent understandings of the borderline personality, particularly the work of Otto Kernberg, he argues that rage-type murderers are victim to primitive defensive processes such as splitting, denial, idealization, devaluation and projective identification. In his words, 'the unconscious denial of affect, and the use of preoedipal defenses in a rigid and controlled personality disorder with dependent and narcissistic features, are pathonomic of catathymia' (Meloy, 1992, p.52).

As is characteristic of borderline pathology, these individuals constantly shift from extreme dependence to feelings of entitlement, from being highly sensitive and easily humiliated to being grandiose about personal capabilities. Meloy makes use of Kernberg's argument, proposing that each object or self-representation carries its own affective charge when cathected. The denial of affect is thus also attached to a particular object relation that has been split off from the rest of the psyche. It is from this split-off affective charge that murderous rage emanates.

The catathymic offender's internal world is split into good and bad objects and all thinking past these polarities becomes unresolvable, creating an internal situation that leads to a build-up of unbearable affect. Along these lines, Meloy

(1992) quotes a patient as saying: 'Either he or I must die, something has to give' (p.58). He believes that verbalizations like this essentially express a wish to annihilate the bad self or object whilst at that moment having no consciousness of the good self or object.

Meloy also finds that these kinds of murderer show clear signs of insecure attachments to significant objects originating from early primary relationships. Because of this, the individual feels bound and controlled by attachments, whilst at the same time fears that significant others will abandon him. For Meloy, this is the prototype of the transference that predisposes the individual to a situation of murder aimed at ending the distress that this dilemma causes. In this way he agrees with Revitch and Schlesinger (1981) that murderous action is propelled by re-enactment.

But why does this escalate into murder? Meloy uses the mechanism of projective identification to explain how this occurs. Earlier, we considered some of the different ways projective identification has been used to understand violent action. For Meloy it is very much about a desperate need for control. In a defensive attempt to protect representations of the self, unwanted bad parts of the self are attributed to an external object, followed by an attempt to control the object. During a period of increasing tension the offender feels more and more vulnerable, and, in an attempt to eliminate feelings of helplessness, he invades the internal object so as to control it or he fears he will be controlled by it. Although a complete breakdown of the boundaries between self and object does not occur, there is growing confusion, because of projection, as to the source of anger, distress and pain. When the confusion is finally located in another person, through projective identification, a sense of magical omnipotent control is exercised over the external object. Finally, 'absolute control of the object as the source of persecutory distress,' Meloy (1992) argues, 'is acted out through violence' (p.62).

It is not clear whether he sees rage murder as having any particular or distinctive dynamic features, as opposed to it simply being an extreme form of escalating violence. He does say, however, that in chronic catathymia, individuals experience conscious fantasies of murder. Although planning of the murder may take place here, it differs from psychopathic motives in that the fantasies are ego-dystonic and are unpleasurable to the person. From a dynamic standpoint, Meloy also views the depression linked to chronic catathymic murder as being a defence against murderous impulses. If external triggers are intense enough, the defence collapses leading to murder.

Finally, Meloy believes that the relief associated with rage murder has two psychological sources. First, it occurs by virtue of the large amount of affect that has been split off through the murder, in phantasy unburdening the self. Second, the relief emerges from the actualization of a fantasized end to a disruptive symbiotic attachment.

Hyatt-Williams: latent murderousness and the indigestible idea of death

In *Cruelty, Violence and Murder*, Hyatt-Williams (1998) discusses over 30 years of experience working with violent prisoners. He agrees with the observation that most rage-type murderers do not show many overt signs of abnormality. But this does not mean that their personalities are free of specific dynamic constellations. 'Despite histories of hitherto apparently blameless lives,' he argues, 'all murderers seem to have a criminal personality' (1998, p.19). For Hyatt-Williams, the 'criminal personality' exists between neurotic and psychotic ways of managing internal experience. Like Meloy, he agrees that borderline dynamics best explain the way these individuals manage experience. The 'criminal' aspect to which he makes reference refers to an entrenched, but often hidden, narcissism. When uncovered, the arrogance of this part of the personality reduces the psychic world to part-objects, in turn dehumanizing the living world that surrounds the potential murderer.

The process of splitting evident in the personality organization he discusses appears to be somewhat different from what is typically associated with the more impulsive, erratic, rapidly cycling borderline personality. He describes a splitting process that is more stable, and perhaps more 'successful', in its effort to keep bad internal experience split off from the rest of the personality.

Hyatt-Williams, at present, provides the most comprehensive account of how defensive organizations operate in rage-type murderers. He draws predominantly from Klein's and Bion's ideas on projective identification, *Ps <->D* interchanges, the container–contained relationship and indigestible mental states. He begins with the premise that we all possess murderous capabilities as manifestations of the death instinct. He argues that it is 'the indigestible idea of death' (p.23) itself that forms the core of this pathological organization which, in turn, constantly threatens psychic development and life-giving processes. Hyatt-Williams calls this 'the death constellation'.

Throughout life, he argues, we continually attempt to work through depressive anxieties related to destructiveness and death, mourning the losses that result. This would also ultimately include mourning the idea of one's own inevitable death. We are ultimately dependent on the containing capabilities of the maternal object to ensure that our own destructiveness acquires a depressive solution where it is mitigated by love and care for the object. In the murderous mind, however, Hyatt-Williams finds that a number of factors force this process into an encapsulated state where 'working through' ceases. He cites a predisposition to excessive envy, the lack of a containing object, exposure to trauma, brutalization and prolonged painful illness as factors that impair the metabolizing process. As a result, associated internal experiences are split off and exist as concrete indigestible objects lying dormant until some external or internal event threatens the status quo. They exist in the form of ideograms, unarticulated images, that are propelled into consciousness when under threat.

The splitting he describes is an attempt to account for why many violent individuals are often described as 'apparently ordinary individuals'. In most cases where destructiveness has not contaminated the whole intrapsychic situation, such as is seen in extreme psychopathy, these individuals possess only a particular area of vulnerability. Here, he is referring specifically to individuals who are suscepti-ble to rage-type murder. In his words:

> There are, however, other persons who have areas of specific vulnerability, but who also possess a healthy part of the personality. In practical terms, unless the area of disturbance that is the Achilles heel is touched upon, one can be reasonably certain that no murderous escalation will occur.
>
> (Hyatt-Williams, 1996, p.35)

To refer back to the case of Ralph; he appeared to be well on his way to a successful career before the murder. He achieved well as a student, had clear ideas about studying law and had a real sense of how to achieve his goals. He was well known and liked as a person and was often described as 'outgoing'. He also did not experience himself as feeling insecure in any way and there was little indication that he suffered regular signs of psychological distress. There is little for us to go on here regarding foreseeing Ralph's murderous propensities. Behind all this, as Hyatt-Williams suggests, rage offenders, like Ralph, hide specific areas of vulnerability.

Hyatt-Williams regards the impact of past trauma, in particular, as causing this kind of specific hypersensitivity in the psyche. Although there was little evidence of this in Ralph's case, it certainly does appear to play a role in some cases. We shall consider this in more detail later. It does seem, however, that hypersensitivity may stem from a number of other factors as well.

One implication of Hyatt-Williams' formulation is that murder is not an inevitability in these individuals. There is no clearly defined plan or motivation to carry it out, despite the presence of the death constellation. Further, his formula-tion, as indicated earlier in his general contribution to understanding violence, places great emphasis on the contemporary environment as to whether explosive murder will take place. Only if circumstances occur in such a way that 'too much happens too soon' and the psyche's digestive capabilities are challenged will these individuals murder. 'Actual murder', he writes, 'takes place when too much pres-sure is experienced by the individual at risk before he or she has had the time, opportunity, or capacity to digest it and detoxicate it psychically' (1998, p.157). The extent to which this situation itself is unconsciously determined by the indi-vidual's prodromal behaviour is unclear in his work. Although rage murder is not premeditated and it is dependent on situational factors, Hyatt-Williams argues that such offenders may experience violent fantasies prior to the murder and thus have some awareness of their own violent propensities.

Owing to the concrete nature of the death constellation, a lack of symbolic capacity is also noted. Its importance in other forms of violence has been discussed earlier. Important here, however, is that a sudden collapse of the symbolic function occurs where symbols turn into symbolic equations. In other words, well-developed symbolic capacity may be evident in that part of the personality prior to the onset of an indigestible situation. This again suggests that disturbance is not always apparent in these individuals.

As a further consequence of the splitting process, murderous action is, according to Hyatt-Williams, 'dynamized by persecutory anxiety' (p.78). Unable to tolerate the psychic pain associated with the encapsulated part of the self, these individuals are susceptible to using powerful forms of projective identification. Here external reality, the victim in this case, becomes the target of the aggressor's unbearable psychic pain. It is externalized then attacked or annihilated in the victim. In what he terms 'the dance of death' (p.21), the unsymbolized fantasy of destroying what is indigestible becomes real, irreversibly changing the external situation.

Hyatt-Williams is in agreement with Meloy on this issue, although he refers to a particular type of projective identification most akin to Bion's (1962a) 'evacuative' type, but with more coherence. In other words, it seldom leads to the chaotic psychosis that Bion describes. Further, its function is most directly about annihilation. In phantasy, this disburdens the self and brings some relief, a point made salient by Wertham and Menninger's early contributions. As Hyatt-Williams points out, however, this process ironically results in further depletion of the self and a diminished ability to deal with stressful life situations. Therefore, ironically, the defensive solution also becomes the vehicle for an escalating vulnerability to act violently.

In keeping with his ideas about violence, the main focus of treatment is aimed at 'restoring psychic digestion and metabolism so there can be learning from life experiences' (p.120). The therapist's containing function is of utmost importance here in facilitating a process of mourning that he observes is absent in the murderer. The capacity to mourn, an essential feature of the depressive position is, in Hyatt-Williams' experience, the main means through which psychic digestion can eventually occur. If successful, it results in reclaiming the ground lost through brutalization. It allows for the restoration of creative life-giving aspects of the psyche and an increased capacity to tolerate psychic pain. However, Hyatt-Williams is not over-optimistic in working with such individuals, claiming that the outcome is either very rewarding or extremely difficult and disappointing. This tends to mirror the deep polarized split that appears to occur in the minds of these offenders. He also argues that, in his experience, extreme acts of destructiveness, like rage murder, can never fully be mourned and at best, treatment can only facilitate an increased maturation of the personality and a move towards a more reparative lifestyle.

FURTHER INVESTIGATIONS

Throughout the previous chapters a number of key problems have been explored related to the psychology of the rage offender. To recapitulate, I have considered the clinical features of the act, pointing out five distinguishing features: dissociation; its affective nature; its motiveless nature; the distinction between chronic and acute catathymia; and finally, particular situational characteristics of the act. We then explored some of the characteristics apparent in the personality of the rage-type murderer evident mainly from criminological and psychological perspectives. This also included reviewing what we know about the evidence of psychopathology in rage-type murder. In essence, I argued that both post-traumatic stress disorder and depression may be associated with rage-type offences and that the dissociation that accompanies the act is not typical of a psychotic disorder. In terms of the general features of the personality, a number of characteristics that approximate a rigidly overcontrolled personality has been outlined. A further trend indicates that these individuals are typically considered to have features of borderline personality disorder. I pointed out, however, that borderline pathology is best seen as encompassing a number of varying personality profiles. With this, I suggested that those who have conceptualized the borderline personality as a dual personality structure appear to describe best the general disposition for the rage-type offender. I also raised a number of questions about the nature of the rage-type murderer's personality, the particular psychodynamic factors involved, and how such factors could be related to 'motiveless' murder.

The formulations of murder presented in this chapter yield an array of theoretical explanations as to why murder occurs in rage-type situations. From an aberrant cathartic act, in earlier formulations, to a more contemporary understanding that such a reaction takes place within a complex field of object relations and personality dynamics. In the later contributions, intrapsychic factors are given different emphasis depending on the author's approach. Meloy, for instance, focuses on the general organization of the personality and the role of attachment, whereas Hyatt-Williams emphasizes the role of the 'death constellation' and the role of trauma.

My own observations are in broad agreement with these more recent formulations. However, a number of questions emerge from this body of work that require further investigation. As we have seen, rage-type offenders are typically non-aggressive, passive and emotionally isolated. All this, however, appears rigorously controlled in a way that makes such individuals appear relatively 'normal'. How are we to understand the underlying psychodynamics of this problem? Related to this, what can be said about the borderline personality organization referred to earlier?

More specifically, if it is agreed that rage murder is ultimately defensive in nature then what is the nature of the defensive organization present here? We have seen how important splitting is as a defence in later formulations of rage murder. But how this operates, or is supported, within the defensive organization is still largely unclear. This raises other questions: is rage characteristic of a particular constellation of object relations that have just been waiting to erupt? Does rage-type murder constitute an enactment? Further, what can be said about the fantasy/phantasy life and representational capacity of these kinds of offender?

Still further, as we have seen, projective identification has been isolated as a key dynamic in violent action. It is used, however, to understand a broad range of behaviours and psychological experiences that have little to do with violent action. Why some forms of projective identification lead to extreme acts like murder is still not clearly understood. Related to this, how should we understand the role the victim plays in the discharge of affect? To what extent might these individuals represent a neglected internal object relationship that is suddenly confronted in reality? Here it becomes just as important to understand how the offender is overwhelmed by a situation, or an object, as it is to understand how the affective discharge itself overwhelms the individual.

In the final part of this book I wish to expand on these questions and others using the dimensions of violence I introduced earlier. It is not only the nature of these dimensions that concern me here; I am also interested in understanding what dimensions best explain the psychodynamic features of rage-type murder and the offender's personality. In doing this, I have prioritized those dimensions that, in my view, appear to hold the most explanatory power.

Part III

Intrapsychic dimensions of rage-type murder

The narcissistic exoskeleton: the defensive organization of the rage-type murderer

Perhaps the most striking observation that has emerged in my work relates to the nature of the defensive organization that is consistently evident in rage-type offenders. For this reason I have given it priority over other dimensions. It also provides the context within which many of the other intrapsychic dimensions can be understood.

Typically, the defensive organization is characterized by a rigid split between a constellation of idealized object relations and internalized bad objects, where the former assumes the position of an outer 'holding' personality. The case of Andrew, a 36-year-old businessman, illustrates this well. I shall draw on this case, as well as others already discussed, to explore these observations further.

ANDREW

Andrew murdered his former business partner by shooting him several times. He hid the body in a shallow grave before eventually giving himself up to the police.

Andrew was the younger of two sons. Although both brothers were fanatical sportsmen, they had little contact during childhood. Andrew's relationship with his father had always been considerably strained. His father was an alcoholic and would often become violent towards his mother when drunk. Several times his mother was hospitalized for her injuries. Andrew recalled witnessing a number of these incidents. From age 6 Andrew also remembered himself and his brother spending long nights having to search the local bars for their inebriated father.

Andrew grew up thinking of his father as a weak and pathetic character. He would often make conscious and unconscious references to his father not feeling like a father to him at all. He wanted no contact with persons like him and rejected everything associated with his father because it was linked to feelings of shame. In his words:

> Thinking back, I was always extremely self-conscious about my father.
> He was pretty pathetic in some ways, in some of the things he did, and

he would feel sorry for himself ... perhaps this is why I have always been anti any kind of aggression, I also don't smoke and have never touched alcohol.

Andrew had always been very close to his mother and often attempted to persuade her to leave his father as he worried about her safety. She did not do this, however, and, although only unconsciously acknowledged, it appears that this led to his losing respect for her too. Whenever he spoke about her, he began by talking about protection and quickly moved on to refer to her as a mother figure who 'could do for herself'. She was not referred to with much emotional warmth. Using some of his words, he relied on her as a 'housekeeper', providing all the 'necessities needed in a home'. Andrew described her as being 'very independent, the breadwinner who could look after herself'. He associated this with his own need for independence and a move away from the family.

During his schooling years Andrew remained very 'independent', which to him meant keeping very much to himself. He developed a keen interest in sport, in which he excelled. His success on the sports field enabled him to pursue a professional career as a sportsman immediately after he had left school. As a result of his sporting achievements he became popular and well known in his community. At this point his life changed a great deal.

In talking about his 'independence' Andrew often made reference to themes linked to turning away from his family, feeling that his movement away made him 'hard' and 'stronger'. He grew in apparent 'willpower' and was 'able to shut things out and carry on'. 'Keeping things in', for Andrew, meant being able to be 'independent'. That he may need love and support was never consciously considered and was strongly linked to a suspicion that his problems would not be believed. It is clear that along these lines his 'independence and success' began to consume his life and there was little else that occupied his mind.

His thoughts about his own needs related to his mother and father were replaced by sporting opportunities and involvements with his 'sporting group' of friends. Andrew talked much about finding ample support in his sporting successes. It suddenly became possible to do most things and he quickly developed a taste for the 'high-life', becoming preoccupied with making sure that he possessed all the necessary symbols of status. Significantly, the people in this world appear to have no depth in terms of how he perceived them. It is rather their ability to reflect his success and preoccupation with material wealth that dominated. He would go to extremes to ensure that people approved of what he did and he spent large amounts of time trying to conform to other people's needs. In his words, he 'became addicted to approval ... I knew that if I was with someone I could be what they wanted, it seemed most important'. Although this pattern of relating occurred across all relationships, he appeared to have maintained better relationships with women.

Andrew married at age 26. He and his wife had two daughters. His business and sporting commitments, however, took up most of his time, leaving little space in his life for his family. Andrew's marriage had virtually collapsed a year prior to the murder, although this did not appear to cause him any great distress or concern at the time. Importantly, his wife knew nothing about the business problems he was going through at the time. His reasons for marriage were most readily associated with the 'successful image' that he found so important to portray. At another level 'family' was also linked to great shame. In his words:

> family, I suppose, says more about who I am really. I know now that family was always difficult for me ... kind of like hard labour in the camps. I felt like a prisoner so I tried to hide it by keeping it separate and hidden ... it made me feel bad though and different from others and kind of embarrassed.

Shortly after his professional sporting career had ended, Andrew began a business selling goods closely linked to the sporting world. After 3 years he decided to take on a partner – a friend and fellow sportsman – to help the business expand. The business ran successfully for a year. Suddenly, however, his partner decided that he wanted to leave the country to pursue a career elsewhere and the business was liquidated. The closure of the business with little warning angered Andrew, but he did not discuss this further with the partner or anyone else. They managed to settle financial matters amicably which essentially led to Andrew taking over the liquidated company's assets. Andrew saw himself as a very trusting person who made business deals with his friends 'on the trust of a handshake'. His trust was broken several times within his 'sporting group' of friends but this significantly brought on few signs of difficulty or distress about maintaining relations with such people. In keeping with this, negative responses from others were mostly avoided or down-played.

Andrew once again set up a similar business on his own that proved to be very successful. Eight months later his previous partner arrived back in the country and wanted a job in Andrew's company as his career prospects had not materialized and he was in need of financial help. Despite Andrew's attempts at convincing him that he did not want to work with him, he persisted. Andrew simply ignored his persistence. A considerable amount of evidence at the trial showed that his partner was known to be very aggressive and had a history of violence.

On the morning of the murder Andrew agreed to meet with his former partner to see if he could settle the matter once and for all. However, the meeting escalated into a heated argument about their past business relationship. Moments later, without hesitation, Andrew shot his former partner several times, killing him instantly. Before the outburst he recalled trying to sit and calm himself but 'felt a deep pain that [he had] never felt before ... something very powerful'. He went on, 'this guy would not leave and he was threatening me, it was all bizarre, like it was not happening'. Andrew had kept a gun at work for 'emergencies'; he had never used it before.

Shocked by what he had done, he tried to revive the man with no success. Soon afterwards he realized the gravity of what he had done and attempted to hide all evidence of the crime. He drove around for several hours with the body in his car not knowing what to do. He decided at that point that he would go to his mother's home and tell her what had happened. Nearing her home, however, he could not bring himself to face her and buried the body in a shallow grave on a plot of land close to where he had played as a child.

It took him a week before he eventually handed himself over to the police and confessed to the murder. During this time it was evident to most around him that he was distressed and had become suicidal.

Andrew had no history of violence whatsoever. He was unaware of being distressed prior to the murder. He reported no conscious thoughts of hurting or killing his victim, nor did he experience any paranoid or obsessional thoughts related to the meeting, prior to the incident. He had, however, been concerned about his own safety as he was aware that this man could became aggressive.

During our sessions together it was important for Andrew to tell me that after the murder his relationship with his father changed significantly. Through his initiation, in his words, 'We were able to have the first conversation we had ever had. It is only now that I can see how much I hated my father.'

The prison authorities described him as a 'quiet hard worker who always tried to do his best for others'. After he was incarcerated he soon gained special privileges for good behaviour.

THE NARCISSISTIC EXOSKELETON

A particular set of object relations appear to stand out in the above case. Most salient is Andrew's conscious identification with an independent, 'successful', all-good object that dominates his interactions once he is able to see himself as separate from his family. Importantly, there is a pressing need evident that these identifications be supported by the admiration of others. There are few signs, however, that these are well defined, emotionally meaningful relationships to him. I came to understand this part of him as being a compensatory defence that was initially associated with an identification with his mother, but was most needed in his move away from needing her. This part of him expressed a need for 'replacement objects' that were more easily accessible and reflected only his success in an idealized way. As we have seen in some of his brief statements about his family, particularly his father, his idealization of particular object relationships was based on the rejection of the 'feeling' and nurturing parts of himself because of their associations with humiliation, aggression and entrapping pain. His 'labour camp' analogy appears to depict this as well as a desperate need to split off any evidence of such pain.

Briefly, in terms of the murder itself, the victim clearly represents a threatening intrusive object, someone who has previously let him down in his business and was threatening his business again. It is this unbearable threat that is most readily linked to his aggressive action. Significantly, his business is strongly linked to his idealized 'successful' identity that, as we shall see, is based on desperate defensive measures.

Much more can be said about the kind of psychic situation that, in effect, unknowingly leads to murder. The presence of a constellation of idealized object relationships appears to be a constant in most cases of rage murder I have explored. Simon, for instance, as we have seen earlier, desperately holds on to the fantasy of an ideal relationship with his wife using various defensive strategies to shield him from the reality of his feelings for her. Ralph, on the other hand, maintains his all-good objects through a perpetual need to identify with a 'negotiating role' that only engages good objects.

The key defensive aim here is to maintain an apparently all-good compliant personality in order to deny and split off intolerable elements of the self that have become associated with badness, weakness or aggression. The compliant part of the personality is characterized by a form of narcissistic relating that appears to be responsible for maintaining this exterior in a rigid but effective manner. The concept of a 'narcissistic exoskeleton' appears to describe best how this outward 'holding' personality functions. This requires some qualification.

It is my contention that this part of the personality, although prominent in appearance, holds little interior psychic space in these offenders. In other words, there is little evidence that this all-good image of the self is a stable part of their internalized object world. Andrew, for instance, shows few signs of being able to maintain this all-good successful part of himself without the constant admiration of his 'sporting group'. He described situations where he would go out of his way to win the approval of others, but once they were unavailable, in his words, 'a sense of hurt and absence would sink in'.

Findings elicited from Thematic Apperception Tests performed on 22 offenders, 9 of whom underwent an intensive interviewing process (Cartwright, 2000), supports this observation by reflecting an internal world dominated by sadness, hurt and isolation that is defended against using idealization. Preoccupation with an ideal good self appears to rely on the immediacy of external objects for its survival. With idealizing objects in close proximity, it appears that their 'sense of goodness' relies more on projective identifications with all-good external objects than it does on a stable internalized part of the self. In this way it appears that projective identification is effectively used to hold idealized good 'outside' the self as a kind of exoskeleton. In our relationship it was apparent to me that Andrew had a pressing need to compare himself with me in terms of status, material wealth and general interests. At first I understood this to be about oedipal rivalry and an attempt to gain supremacy over me. But on closer scrutiny the way he related to me appeared to serve a different purpose. It seemed that his pressing need was more about locating parts of me that he could project into. In doing so he was able to identify parts of himself in me which he could then idealize and further hope for my admiration in return. An important implication of this process was the suspension of any real exploration of his difficulties. I had been drawn into an idealizing interaction that he needed if he was to maintain a sense of security that, in turn, shielded him from parts of himself that were felt to be unmanageable.

I use the term 'narcissistic exoskeleton' for two reasons. First, the external objects that form part of the system have a narcissistic quality to them. They are invested, in phantasy, with parts of the offender's self, and the distinction between self and the external object's needs, feelings and motivations are blurred. 'Narcissistic' also refers to a propensity towards the fantastical *creation* of internal objects as a means of denying pain (Rosenfeld, 1987). Second, the image of an exoskeleton best depicts the nature of this structure as being situated outside, or on the periphery of, the self, enclosing an interior.

An exoskeleton has a dual function which parallels the kind of object relations evident in rage offenders. It both supports and contains an internal structure whilst simultaneously protecting it from outside threats, much like a rigid sheet of armour. To return to Andrew. He attempts to abandon his established internal objects through creating new identifications which are typified by an idealized form of independence based on sporting achievements. These form the basis of the exoskeletal structure, hiding an interior that can no longer have contact with the external world. At the same time, the vulnerable interior is protected from the threats of the outside world. As is my observation with most cases, Andrew is preoccupied with searching for confirmations of an idealized good world in other external objects in order to uphold the defensive structure.

It appears that the rigidity of this defensive system goes some way to explain why rage-type offenders are often described as apparently stable, an issue we explored earlier in considering the role of mental illness and salient personality characteristics in the propensity to commit explosive violence. Not only does the split between an idealized exterior and internalized bad objects grant an appearance of 'normality', its defensive and controlling nature appears to explain how symptomatology synonymous with distress and conflict are more readily suppressed in these cases. Here, an acknowledgement of suffering and symptoms of distress is linked with a chain of associated unbearable ideas characterized by incapacity, weakness and badness. This dynamic, one might argue, is a common feature found in many cases where denial and acute defensiveness are key factors. What is peculiar to these kinds of offender, however, is the extreme danger associated with weakness and vulnerability that, in turn, gives rise to a hypertrophied defensive system that inhibits the awareness of signs of distress and its symptomatic expression. 'I never get depressed', Andrew told me once, 'sometimes I get a little sad but it only lasts a little while because I force myself to think of the good things that I have done and I also think of God'.

The idealized object system varies across cases depending on the specific characteristics of the objects involved, but it appears that the essential structure and function remains a key feature. The self is identified with an all-good object world that constantly maintains itself through cycles of relatively benign projective identifications with external objects. Here, projective identifications are used to enlist collusively the support of external objects in fostering a 'belief' in this perception of the self. The projections do not appear to be evacuative or intrusive in nature in the sense that they are 'forced' into external objects (Bion, 1962a). Evidence from case histories and my psychotherapeutic experience with such offenders suggests that this is mostly achieved through appeasing and constantly satisfying the object, a strategy that maintains the image of an all-good self and, at the same time, avoids any potential conflict. We see this with Andrew where he never addresses hurt or conflict within himself. He avoids this simply by adopting the other's position on the matter. In time, he was able to develop some insight into this way of relating. In his words, 'I strove to be like everyone else. In that way I could never really be singled out or feel that something was wrong.' Similarly, Simon spent much time describing the importance of constantly worrying about his wife and making sure she was always happy. If she was not he would immediately try to remedy the situation by doing whatever she wanted in a submissive manner. Alternatively, if she did anything wrong, even in terms of the love affair she had, Simon would quickly 'forgive' her and attempt to do more for her in order to maintain his 'ideal world' perception.

In some cases, however, the perpetuation of this veil of goodness is also maintained through a rigidly held self-righteous, and sometimes attacking, attitude towards objects not perceived to reflect the ideal self. Here, righteousness renders such an individual particularly difficult to engage with owing to a constant adherence to perceived expectations and 'rules' that are used to justify actions. This was clearly apparent in a particularly difficult therapy I conducted with a man who had attacked a number of people at his workplace after being informed that he needed to increase his productivity. Here was a man who did 'everything right and by the book' with an overzealous adherence to the rules of the workplace to the point that it was very difficult to fault him on anything. Similarly, the transference was dominated by a preoccupation with 'doing things right' and a persistent need to know what the 'rules' of therapy were.

Once he had made up his mind about what I 'wanted' from him in therapy, he busied himself with making sure that he adhered to these perceived needs. In other words, he began to create an exoskeleton that made sure it would be very difficult to get to know parts of him that were not built on what he perceived me to want. On the occasions when I attempted to challenge this and show him how this paralleled his behaviour elsewhere, he would become very defensive and attacking in his approach. He would constantly repeat his claims that he was only doing what he was told to do and argued that I was being unfair and deceptive, in turn, disowning any responsibility for the process. Later, his defensiveness shifted to attacking 'negative feelings' he perceived me to have towards him. In his righteous manner he claimed that I was not being fair and sticking to the rules of therapy that 'were about supporting and affirming' him. In short, he was attacking parts of me that exposed him to a deep sense of shame because my interpretations no longer supported his defensive strategy – the narcissistic exoskeleton.

The interaction of the ideal self with other objects is similar to Kohut's (1978) description of the *mirroring* and *idealizing transferences* he found to be present in narcissistic patients. Earlier, in considering some of the features of rage, we saw how this kind of interaction can be linked to a need to maintain control over the environment in order to prevent narcissistic injury and the sudden loss of self-esteem. Kohut's understanding, however, does not appear to explain adequately the rigidity of this system and how active the individual is in manipulating his objects to maintain narcissistic reflection. Here, the mechanism of projective identification is more instructive where good objects are held 'outside' the self in order to maintain the split between internalized badness and idealized parts of the self. This is somewhat different from more typical uses of pathological forms of projective identification where bad experience is usually projected outwards.

In its non-pathological form, projective identification is the mechanism through which communication occurs between mother and infant (Bion, 1962a). In this process the projection of part of the self into another is contained and returned in a modified form to be used for further emotional and mental growth. This does not seem to operate in the cases isolated here as the cycles of projection are not muta-tive or able to nourish the individual's internal world in any way. They are simply repetitive and self-fulfilling. Andrew aptly uses the word 'addiction' to describe his compulsive need to set things up so that he could read some degree of affirma-tion into almost everything. To refer to another case, Ralph continuously involves himself in 'negotiating activities' in an attempt to perpetuate an image of himself as all-good. He benefits from this as long as the negotiations are successful, but breaks contact when the situation becomes difficult and conflicted. Both Andrew and Ralph display little tolerance if the object does not simply return what is projected, expressing little desire, conscious or otherwise, to be changed by the external object. Thus no change or emotional growth can occur here. The strategy becomes self-fulfilling, essentially serving a defensive function. Ralph's own astonishment in not being able to grasp why the 'negotiating role' was so impor-tant to him also suggests that the role fulfils a defensive need and is not a source of mental stimulation or growth.

A similar process occurs when the offender is the recipient of bad experience or intolerable projected states. In many cases there are indications of bad experience simply being denied or immediately covered up by the ideal good self, giving the impression it has been dealt with, or that the offender is left unaffected by the incident. In Andrew's case, he is unable to deal with the true impact of his business partner's desertion. He denies the real implications and consequences of this and turns to rationalizations related to 'always trusting in a good outcome, no matter what'.

Often, there is a consistent theme of bad, aggressed and conflictual aspects of the self being denied. Because of this there is usually a reluctance to engage in any behaviours associated with aggression, even when defensive or adaptive. Anything associated with aggression, even assertiveness in many cases, is associ-ated with 'badness' and split off.

It is difficult to understand Andrew's actions after the murder especially because there was no criminal motive evident. Our thinking here can only be speculative. It is most probable, however, in the context of his split object relations, that his actions were propelled by disbelief in his own aggression and the need to get rid of everything it – the bad-object system – represented in a very concrete way. The fact that he also buried the body in a place directly associated with his childhood also intrigued me. Listening to his associations here, I came to understand this to be part of an attempt to put the seeds of his violent actions back where they belonged, in fantasy, undoing the murder. Again, this appeared to be consistent with his defensive style.

Three years after the murder, when I first met Andrew, there were already signs that the split between the idealized 'independent self' and the 'bad self' had been worked on internally. He was able to relate to his own aggression and the original rejecting object relationship with which it was associated. I understood his courage in re-establishing contact with his father to be a clear indication of this. Andrew also reported a short dream that appeared to indicate some move towards depressive experience. He reported the dream as follows:

> I and my wife were in a long queue waiting to order take-away pizza. We were about to be served and this guy who was in a hurry kept on nudging me, you know, to move along. Eventually I stood back and said please go and get your pizza, I will wait.

His associations suggested that the nudging man represented a 'hurrying hungry person' who had the potential to get angry if he did not get his own way. Thoughts about himself represented in the dream related to a desperate wish to be with his wife. He wanted to do things differently and not 'rush around in order to make myself feel good'. The dream appeared to portray the emergence of a more adaptive defensive style that was also evident in the transference. We understood the dream in two meaningful ways. First, it seemed to represent an adaptive repetition of the crime scene where Andrew overcomes his anxiety and accommodates for the intrusion or threat in a non-violent way. Second, the two figures in the dream also appeared to represent two historically different parts of himself. The first is strongly associated with the part of himself that is 'hungry' for self-affirmation and more vulnerable to violent action – 'nudging' – if obstacles are placed in the way. The second appears to signify a more adaptive self more able to tolerate distress because of his concern for other objects.

It is worth noting that in many cases the narcissistic exoskeleton does not simply lead to the denial of conflict; a kind of pseudo-digestion of the conflict also occurs. Here, there may be some acknowledgement of hostility, betrayal or the like. But they leave the individual unmoved, unaffected, often giving the outward appearance that the problem has been dealt with. All indications are, however, that it remains undigested in the psyche and is allocated to a 'bad self' in order to salvage the ideal self and the apparent normality that it portrays. I shall return to this shortly in discussing the borderline personality.

Thus far we have explored the idealized good-object system prominent in most offenders. What, however, is the nature of the 'bad self' that results from identifications with bad internalized objects? In most cases it remains split-off and dormant in the personality, protected by the all-good object system. With Andrew, the trauma of witnessing his father's repeated abuse is split off and associated with all men, preventing any meaningful contact. Prior to the murder, there are few signs that the abuse and its consequences were ever consciously acknowledged – they remained suspended in the psyche like concrete indigestible objects. It was surprising that Andrew had never given any thought to how his father's behaviour had led to a total rejection of alcohol and other things he perceived to represent his father. This only occurred to him in talking it through with me. It appears that interaction with the world had been restricted as a consequence of avoiding confrontation with this part of himself represented in external objects. Instead, Andrew interacted mainly with women and even then, they were represented as one-dimensional objects within a defensive system that used them to bolster the split between good and bad objects.

Steiner's (1993) concept of a 'psychic retreat' depicts a similar internal problem. He uses the term to describe a particular internal structure where relief is sought through a withdrawal from any meaningful contact with others because it is felt to be too threatening. The withdrawal forms an encapsulated system that remains isolated and stagnant. In some cases the system of defences brings substantial relief and, as a result, is often idealized as a haven free of conflict. But alongside this some parts of the self are felt to be persecutory or 'deadly'. Although a similar dynamic occurs in the cases I have explored, it is not the retreat itself that is idealized but the pseudo-enriching contact that occurs between self and external objects.

Fairbairn's (1952) idea that the infant internalizes bad object relations as a defensive manoeuvre, as discussed earlier, appears to be particularly relevant in understanding the narcissistic exoskeleton. He believed that the internalization of bad objects serves, in fantasy, to 'remove' the bad object from the external world thus saving good object relations from its destructive influence. The internalization process is also an attempt to bring the bad object under the control of the self. In Fairbairn's formulation, however, the internalized bad object then dominates the personality through attacking libidinized object relations. This dynamic is not usually apparent in rage-type offenders. It is more typically observable in aggressive borderline patients and found in its extreme in the psychopathic personality where destructive narcissism (Rosenfeld, 1987) dominates psychic functioning. Here, bad objects are idealized, forming gangs or systems that work to attack good nurturing object relations. In rage offenders the internal 'attacking' or aggressive dynamic is not reversed in this way. Although the articulation or engagement of the 'bad self' with other parts of the internal world is minimal, when it is evident in the analysis, the 'attack' takes place in the opposite direction. The dominant, or righteous, good self attacks the damaged 'feeling' part of the self that has become assimilated into the bad-object system.

Sometimes the 'bad self' exists in a stable projected form long before the actual attack itself, where the murder victim is perceived to be an all-bad attacking object. There may, of course, be some reality to such a perception and this would depend on the nature of the case. But often such a perception is magnified because it is needed to maintain the split between good and bad objects. I was made aware of this process in working with a man I was seeing for psychotherapy to help him with his anger that had, on one occasion, led to serious violence towards his wife. His marriage was particularly conflictual and, from what I could gather, his wife was clearly quite abusive towards him. As the transference–countertransference inter-action unfolded, however, it emerged that he had a vested interest in his wife being a bad aggressive object, leaving him constantly victimized. Once he had found a way to make me the abusive object – my silence was seen as abusive in this instance – he had room for his next manoeuvre: to justify, in a righteous way, that he was the good party in the conflict. It formed part of a phantasy that left him free of having to identify a bad internal object within himself. This appeared to contribute to the entrapping nature of the relationship observed in this case where the offender displayed a chronic inability to deal with the situation by walking away from conflict in order to re-engage the problem constructively. It is entrap-ping because the offender has an unconscious vested interest in the victim contin-uing to play the role of an all-bad attacking object. I do not wish to undermine the reality of the difficult situations such abused persons find themselves in here, but only mean to explore how the defensive system may also be invested in this reality. I view the impact of such abuse as being an important determinant of violence in its own right and, to this end, it shall be explored as a separate dimension in the next chapter.

In most cases, however, there are few indications that the bad-object system is projected in this way, perhaps supporting Weiss *et al.*'s (1960) finding that explosive offenders are unable to use projection as a 'successful' defence. To recall, they hypothesized that projective mechanisms were not used because they leave the individual feeling swamped by bad objects, further reminding him of his own inadequacies. Certainly, in the immediacy of the act of violence, a massive projection of intolerable bad objects appears to occur, but this is due to a sudden rupturing of the defensive system and not part of the action of the defensive system itself.

For most then, the 'bad self' remains concealed and held in behind the narcis-sistic exoskeleton. Returning to Fairbairn (1952), what appears to emerge here is an accumulation of bad experience that remains unmodified and is prevented, in most cases, from gaining some relief via projection. If one accepts that the offender's personality is essentially dominated by the perpetual 'creation' of idealized good objects, unfettered by any bad objects, then the problem with the projection of bad experience appears understandable. Therefore, from a slightly different perspective from that of Weiss and his colleagues, it is also likely that the projection of the 'bad self' would run the risk of contaminating the ideal world they have, in phantasy, created. In this way, the separation between 'external' and 'internal' – the exoskeleton and the interior – as corresponding representations of idealized good objects and all-bad objects, is important to maintain.

How should we understand the implications and consequences of this good/bad, external/internal, split? I have found it most useful to see it in terms of a suspension of the *Ps <-> D* process of psychic digestion. Although he does not refer to it specifically as psychic digestion, Bion (1962a) introduces this model to illustrate the constant oscillations that occur in the psyche between splitting 'paranoid' processes (*Ps*) and integrative depressive processes (*D*). According to him, all emotional and mental processes continually oscillate in this way in order to accommodate new material and create 'new thoughts'. Thus thoughts and emotions undergo a splitting process and thereafter couple together in a different way provided the individual can contain such a process. This, however, appears to be retarded in most rage offenders where the defensive organization interrupts and polarizes the process. Here, interchange between *Ps* and *D* is suspended and bad objects remain unmetabolized. The bad-object system exists in an encapsulated state and consists mainly of paranoid experience, in the Kleinian sense of the word, that cannot achieve temporary resolution in the depressive position.

It is tempting, following Wertham (1937) and some of the other earlier formulations discussed previously, to conclude that the accumulation of undigested bad experience is what ultimately leads to a cathartic explosion when it becomes intolerable. Viewed in this way, the attack or murder is perpetrated by the 'bad self' when it bursts through all psychological defences. As we have seen, this certainly appears correct when applied to the phenomenology of explosive rage. However, the situational factors evident here and the acts of rage murder that I have reconstructed appear to indicate that the mechanism of action is somewhat different. We shall return to this in discussing how some of the other intrapsychic dimensions of violence contribute to the act of rage-type murder.

The defensive organization observed in these offenders bears some similarities to a number of other formulations. Wertham (1962) notes a kind of arrogance in the personality of the catathymic offender that lies in opposition to extreme inadequacy, fear of incompetence and passivity. This appears similar to the split found to be evident here. Arrogance is perhaps a useful description of the ideal good self, typified by a conscious attitude in the individual of being able to tolerate anything that comes his or her way.

The defensive organization also bears a resemblance to Winnicott's (1965) notion of the False and True Self. The False Self emerges when the mother 'repeatedly fails to meet the infant gesture; instead she substitutes her own gesture which is to be given sense by the compliance of the infant' (p.145). Later, he describes the situation as follows: 'When the mother's adaptation is not good enough at the start the infant might be expected to die physically, because cathexis of external objects is not initiated. The infant remains isolated. But in practice the infant lives, but only falsely'(p.146). In a similar way the narcissistic exoskeleton and the False Self maintain a defensive system through compliance with the external world. According to Winnicott, through compliance with the mother, or environmental demands, the False Self defensively hides True Self potential. It is hidden because it has become associated with 'unthinkable anxiety' that is due mainly to maternal neglect. It is likely that this kind of primitive anxiety is also associated with the hidden 'bad self' in the above formulation.

For Winnicott, such individuals lack an ability to nurture and sustain mental objects or make use of internal resources. The fate of the True Self is ultimately restricted to bodily sensation and is not able to gain representational space in the psyche. This manifests in experiences of emptiness, isolation and boredom. In a similar way, in the process of psychotherapy, once rage offenders have become aware of how they use the protective exoskeleton as a defence, they are often confronted with a sense of empty indecision and boredom. Here they face a desperate struggle with a very real sense of meaninglessness attached to their own actions and behaviours.

The term 'False Self', however, carries with it the connotation that it is simply defensive and makes no real contribution to the individual's development. As Glasser (1997) points out, whilst the False Self may be compliant, this should be interpreted not only as a useless, empty part of the self. He believes that the False Self is capable of being quite a functional part of the personality and also serves to protect others from the individual's aggression. Indeed, we have seen this in many of the offenders I have discussed thus far. Most are reasonably successful as a result of False Self activity. This is so until they are forced, by internal and external factors, to confront split-off parts of the self.

Referring to the False Self and its association with apparent normality, Glasser (1996) suggests that some violent individuals display a greater propensity for 'simulation'. In his words, simulation is 'a defensive process in which the individual *appears* to develop qualities or features which are valued by the person to whom he or she is in relation' (p.278). Glasser seems to be referring more to the psychopathic personality here, where this process is conscious and deliberately deceptive. Although not typically psychopathic, 'simulation' also appears to operate in rage offenders where over-compliant parts of the narcissistic exoskeleton attempt to guard against destructive impulses. The over-compliance and over-obliging nature of these individuals, most readily observed in the transference, best illustrates the kind of 'simulation' that occurs here. I have already referred to such a case in considering a patient's desperate attempts to comply with the 'rules' of therapy. Here, his attempts at simulation could be seen in his persistent efforts to mimic my therapeutic manner and what he perceived to be expected in the process.

This is similar to what Gaddini (1992) has referred to as 'imitation', a primitive form of identification that will be discussed further when considering the offenders' capacities for object-relating. Suffice it to say here that Glasser's concept is formulated as being associated with a bad destructive part of the personality, whereas in my formulation it appears more aligned with the good compliant self.

The similarities between the above defensive organization and Deutsch's (1942) description of the 'as if' personality are also important to note. The 'as if' personality is characterized by 'disavowal', the denial of the realistic significance of things. This differs greatly, however, from the more psychotic obliteration of reality. Deutsch claims that the inability truly to engage the realistic qualities of the object has the advantage of ensuring a conflict-free psychic reality that makes the individual appear 'as if' he or she leads a 'normal' unproblematic existence. Although such individuals are able to show apparent emotional, sensitive capacities, she finds that a closer analysis reveals that they display a marked absence of inner experience. The narcissistic exoskeleton shares similar characteristics. It has been formulated as disavowal of the realistic nature of 'badness' in the object in order to uphold an 'as if' engaging interaction, with an all-good object. As is the case in Deutsch's formulation, this part of the offenders' interaction however, lacks any clearly defined representational or psychic space. We have understood this to be the consequence of a defensive split between bad objects that occupy internal space, whilst the all-good objects are 'kept alive' by keeping them, in phantasy, 'outside' the internal world.

The division, or stand-off, between 'internal' and 'external' reality is further supported by Britton's (1998) recent formulation of the 'as if' personality. Although not relating this defensive organization to violence, he views the split as a consequence of the individual feeling unable truly to engage internal or external reality as both appear equally terrifying. The only option, therefore, is to 'exist' on the borderline between the two. In this state the individual may appear very well adjusted, with the stand-off also serving a pseudo-containing function for the individual. In reality, Britton argues, such individuals can only maintain this defensive strategy by enduring a passive existence and by suspending all belief in self and others. This resonates in a particular way with my observations. On the one hand, the internal world is dominated by the bad-object system, making internal experience dangerous and unavailable. On the other hand, real engagement with external objects is equally dangerous as the ambiguous good and bad nature of real objects threatens to disrupt the defensive strategy that strives to keep bad experience, and its specific associations with shame and aggression, out of their perceived external reality. In other words, this part of the psyche displays little tolerance for depressive experience.

But how does the defensive predisposition outlined here compel an individual to commit murder? Although this would also depend on other factors still to be discussed, there are indications that rage-type murder takes place when narcissistic defences are breached, exposing the 'bad self' in a way that can no longer be tolerated. The situation triggers an internal crisis whereby this part of the self is, in phantasy, evacuated and destroyed in the external object. This is in accordance with Batemen's (1998) understanding that violence is more likely to occur in narcissistic organizations when there is a sudden shift in the defensive system. The details of the act itself will be discussed further once all intrapsychic dimensions have been explored.

Borderline Personality Organization

We have already concluded, based on previous research, that borderline personality disorder has often been implicated in rage crimes. Earlier, we also considered two different types of borderline functioning, one more stable than the other. The question remains: does the defensive system discussed here constitute a borderline personality organization? Clearly, the rigidity of the defensive organization does not fit the typical impulsive and unstable borderline pattern that typifies *The Diagnostic and Statistical Manual IV*'s (American Psychological Association, 1994) diagnostic classification of borderline personality disorder. This is not to say that such individuals are not capable of committing rage attacks. As pointed out earlier, the impulsive borderline pattern has been previously implicated in rage-type offences by a number of authors (Satten *et al.*, 1960; Meloy, 1992; Kernberg, 1992; Millon, 1996). Here, the ego remains fickle and regressed, collapsing in the face of minor frustrations and manifesting in impulsive antisocial behaviours. But the particular group of offenders I am interested in shows few signs of being impulsive in this way. Significantly, violent individuals who do fit the more impulsive and unstable pattern differ from the rage offenders I am referring to in two ways: first, in the former, there is often a conscious identification with the 'bad self', resulting in a perversion of object relations. The 'bad self' becomes omnipotent and powerful and aims to destroy good nurturing objects. This is essentially the reverse of what I have described earlier. Second, the more impulsive types usually have a history of minor violent acts and they are often manipulative in threatening violence. Given this, violence is more predictable and is often provoked by the offender in some way.

I proposed, in discussing the borderline organization earlier, that the more impulsive profile may simply be a regressed presentation of the *overcontrolled* personality often observed in rage-type offences. Although this may occur, some individuals display a long history of unstable impulsive behaviours suggesting that the controlled exterior held in place by the narcissistic exoskeleton does not dominate the defences used here. Although sharing similar borderline defensive strategies – splitting, idealization, denial and projective identification – the defensive system I have explored is synonymous with a more controlled borderline organization.

With similar concerns, Gallwey (1985) outlines two different dual-personality profiles that fall within the broad category of borderline personality organization. His formulations are worth mentioning in some detail here as they clarify some of the dynamic differences observed in borderline personalities that are vulnerable to pathological forms of aggression. His work also supports observations made here about the 'narcissistic exoskeleton'.

Gallwey bases his formulations on Bion's ideas about a split personality organization. Importantly, as he observes, if conceptualized in this way, regression need not be used to explain the expression of primitive defences because the personality functions as two separate systems, one able to function independently of the other.

In the first type of dual personality, the more impulsive profile, the pseudo-self serves to conceal deficiencies caused in the ego by prolonged infantile trauma. As a result a large part of the ego remains in a regressed state. These individuals are intolerant of separation experiences and are plagued by feelings of hopelessness and profound loss. The ego, however, remains somewhat functional through the use of various strategies. Most evident is the use of primitive fantasies to control objects, which set up a parasitic dependence on 'host' objects to maintain this illusion of normality. The illusion of control may also be maintained by reversing the problem of dependency, making objects dependent on the self. Gallwey argues that aggression resulting from 'emotional hunger and sense of poverty' (p.135) is mostly dealt with through addictive behaviours. He goes on to say, in these individuals 'vengeful feelings cannot find legitimate expression, this may lead to compliant, passive, even masochistic relationships with others' (p.135). He does not, however, make it clear why these vengeful feelings cannot be directly expressed.

The expression of aggression and other antisocial behaviours in this personality organization form part of the defensive system that strives to maintain the fickle ego. For this reason, according to Gallwey, these individuals often appear intimidating and frightening to others. They 'have a clear tendency to collapse in the face of almost any hazard or frustration, are usually unable to sustain an independent existence, show frequent bouts of self-destructiveness, are almost continually manipulative and self-preoccupied, and are generally poorly contained individuals' (p.135).

Gallwey argues that most habitual offenders fit this personality profile and are most vulnerable to committing acts of homicide when there is a threat of the loss of an object. The violence is thus a defensive attempt to preserve his dependency on the object. He argues that in cases such as this 'violent behavior can be as much a desperate attempt to establish some supportive link with an object of over-dependency as [it is] an expression of pure destructiveness' (p.136).

Gallwey's second dual personality appears closer to the mark in outlining a more 'stable', but also more explosive, profile. The individual has a more coherent ego but this can only be maintained as long as it is split off from a more destructive and disturbed area of the personality. If this is successful, such individuals may live reasonably fulfilling lives. The encapsulated part of the personality, in Gallwey's opinion, consists of '"undigested" memories or primitive images built of experiences connected with being terrorized or exposed to excessive pain or brutality through non-accidental injury' (p.147). If this is disrupted through some form of vulnerability it triggers a catastrophic discharge of violent emotions. Because of an extraordinary capacity to maintain the split between these two separate systems, the discharge of these primitive affects is usually brief and circumscribed. They appear relatively stable and there is little evidence of any deterioration in their personality after violent acts. Further, according to Gallwey, overt psychotic symptoms are rarely detected.

Consistent with my observations, he argues that extreme forms of encapsulation may explain why such offenders show few signs of distress. He describes them as shy and passive with some neurotic features. Because they are so often free of any gross symptomatology, he finds that organic causes are often sought in an attempt to explain their aberrant violence, despite there being no evidence of this. Although these individuals may appear 'normal', the deeply entrenched splitting process inevitably leads to an impoverished personality structure as much psychic energy is spent internally on maintaining the split.

Gallwey also claims that the offence 'often has bizarre, violent and quasi-sexual features' (p.142) and, at times, there may be evidence of a sexual perversion or non-habitual delinquency, despite the individual being socially well adjusted. In my experience, however, this is not a typical or defining feature of the rage-type offender. In most cases, the rigid appeasing nature of their defensive style does not allow such sexualization to occur (see Chapter 8).

For the most part, however, I think Gallwey's second dual-personality formulation, combined with the concept of the 'narcissistic exoskeleton', sheds some light on the internal dynamics of Megargee's (1966) original concept of the *overcontrolled* offender which, earlier, I associated with the borderline personality. In this chapter I have essentially argued that 'overcontrol' has its source in a system of defences which rigorously control split-off aspects of the self by establishing an idealized 'exoskeleton' that denies and controls the existence of the 'bad self'. I have tried to show that the defensive structure is fundamentally interpersonal in nature and based on interaction with external objects. Understood in this way, the idea that 'holding things in' until violence eventually erupts is not an accurate explanation of what occurs at an intrapsychic level. The defensive system is made up of a web of intrapsychic and interpersonal correlates that work together not so much to 'hold things in', but to desperately hold on to an idealized shield that renders the self 'quietly' invincible. This is so, of course, until some obstacle threatens to expose the bad-object system.

The question of chronicity

One final problem needs to be addressed before we proceed to other dimensions of rage-type murder. In attempting to understand the impact this kind of defensive organization has on the offender's murderous behaviour, we cannot avoid questions regarding the chronicity of these defences. By definition, defensive organizations are fixed and enduring parts of the personality that prevent growth or learning from experience (Spillius, 1988; Steiner, 1993). But how can we be sure that these rigid means of organizing experience predispose such offenders to explosive violence? This is especially the case given that the majority of offenders referred to here were treated or assessed after the crime. Given the trauma associated with the murder and all the implications it has for the offender, surely the construction of an idealized defensive self is an effective means of dealing with unbearable psychic pain *after* the murder? In other words, how do we know that these defences are not simply a consequence of the murder? This is very difficult to ascertain and indeed is a problem with all *ex post facto* forms of analyses.

There are, however, two factors that support the claim that my analysis picks up on enduring defensive patterns. The first simply draws on the theory in this area claiming that defensive organizations are deeply rooted in the personality and require considerable psychic work if they are to change in some way. Whilst traumatic experience may rupture defensive patterns, it is unlikely that the defensive system would be entirely transformed by the murder and all its implications. The second factor refers to collateral sources that were used to substantiate my interpretive findings. In most cases, as was the case with Andrew, I used material available from court reports as well as information from significant others who knew the offender prior to the crime. In other words, my interpretation of intrapsychic processes discussed here is also based on historical reports of enduring behaviours in the individual's past. Certainly, material from therapy sessions and interviews is inevitably subject to a process of 'narrative smoothing' (Spence, 1982) by both the offender and myself. Nevertheless, most of the evidence that supports the idea that these character patterns existed prior to the murder could be corroborated by court reports.

Chapter 7

Representational capacity, internal objects and situational factors

What can be said about the nature of other intrapsychic dimensions of violence? There are a number of significant psychic events that help us further understand what lies behind the explosive nature of the act, its motiveless nature and other clinical features as outlined earlier. It appears that a particular part of the personality has impoverished representational abilities that are more vulnerable to collapse in the face of threat. When this occurs mental action is suddenly equated with physical action. Part of this vulnerability may also result from the offender's predisposition to act out of a symbiotic position. Here, symbiotic object relations are very closely adhered to for the purpose of self-definition but, at the same time, are also dangerously entrapping. Finally, we shall consider how the offender's internal world parallels, and is in interaction with, many aspects of the external situation. I shall use the case of Grant, an offender I saw in psychotherapy 3 years after he had committed his crime, to illustrate my broader observations regarding the aforementioned dimensions.

GRANT

Grant, a 38-year-old teacher, shot and killed his wife and 5-year-old daughter after his wife had insulted him for not doing a household task that she had asked him to do.

Grant came from a family of five. He was the middle child, with a brother 4 years his senior and a sister 2 years younger. His father was a successful store manager and his mother a housewife. Grant's upbringing was unproblematic: his parents were described as very caring, at times 'spoiling' him. Although no overt conflict between Grant and his father was reported, his father was largely absent during his early and teenage years. His father worked late hours, often spending days away from home, leaving Grant with a sense that he had never had the opportunity to get to know his father. He hardly mentioned his father during our time together. Apart from this, the family appeared extremely close and family members would often spend time together. Grant was especially close to his mother. He talked about her in a highly idealized way and she was often associated with an endless ability to provide for others. Through his eyes his mother was extremely cooperative and obliging, and there was little that she was not capable of. She was also associated with creating a place of safety for him.

The central narrative that emerged across most of our sessions together was about a boy who grows up in an extremely 'supportive' and good family. His mother 'spoils' him by allowing him to do 'adult things' and there is no sense of any negative or difficult experience in the family. Despite this, he feels that he cannot reveal all of himself to them and has to do secretly things that are associated with 'his own thoughts'. He is quiet but can open up more to his mother. She, like no other, becomes a measure of his self-esteem. He manages best to do this by being obliging and restrictive in his behaviours. In Grant's words:

> No matter what I do my mother is always in my thoughts, no matter what ... I listen to them [the thoughts] most of the time because she is always right and so I follow her and get rewards. Sometimes it meant not doing certain things because she wanted to do something. Some people, including my wife, thought that it was very strange because I would want to be there all the time. She [his wife] was mad once because we didn't go on holiday one year because my mother didn't want it.

Grant trained to be a teacher immediately after he had finished high school. It was here that he first met his future wife. From the outset, their parents were not happy with the relationship as the pair came from different religious backgrounds. He made no attempt to deal with these problems despite his parent's willingness to discuss them. Instead, they eloped and were married in that same year.

Soon afterwards problems in their marriage started. His wife was reported to have become abusive towards him for petty reasons, such as his coming home slightly late from work and wanting to go and visit his family. They had one daughter together but soon got divorced because he could no longer tolerate his wife's anger which, at times, would turn into violence – she had kicked or slapped him on some occasions. By all accounts she could be very volatile and had been to see a number of doctors about the problem. After one such incident, Grant went back to live with his parents. Shortly afterwards they were divorced but he remarried her only a few months later. The trouble continued, however, and this pattern repeated itself with them getting divorced for a second time. Once again he remarried her, claiming that he felt responsible for his daughter and also believed that he still loved his wife and needed her.

Grant spoke of his wife as being both extremely good and caring, on the one hand, and abusive and violent on the other. When his wife was violent he felt he could never hit back or push her away in defence. In his words, ' I just never had it in me ... Besides that, I would calm her and she would love me again, that's how it always was.' This kind of behaviour was also motivated by an overstated concern about others hearing them or knowing that something was wrong. As reward for these efforts, most people around him saw them as a 'perfect loving couple'.

As we have seen, Grant tried to escape her violence several times by separating from her, but was always drawn back by his myopic focus on 'her ability to love with everything'. Ironically, when he was apart from her, he found that he often encountered fears that something, or someone bad and abusive, would enter his life if he did not go back to her. He felt, in his words, 'dependent and drawn in by her good heart'. On another occasion he expressed it as follows: 'It's crazy that I went back isn't it? But I went back because I wanted everything to be perfect in the name of how she would love me and make me feel ... that made everything disappear.' The romanticized 'perfect' dreams he had, before and after the murder, about his wife also appear related to this theme. For example, he dreamt once, before the murder, of his wife sitting on a throne eating lavish foods whilst he anxiously made sure the foods were available for her.

Grant would also often talk in an idealized manner about other parts of his life such as his parents and his religious faith. Despite this, I was struck by the difficulty he had in elaborating on his thoughts and feeling about these issues. He struggled to describe his parents to me despite my attempts to support him and could not get past simple isolated words like 'nice' and 'wonderful' to describe them. This left me with no clear image of them in my own mind. It should be said that there were no indications here that he was actively resisting such attempts.

Grant's difficulty in 'thinking along with me', or elaborating on his thoughts, became even more apparent when I began to pick up on possible areas of conflict and inconsistencies in some of his statements. He became agitated and struggled to elaborate on these elements in any way. Once, perhaps at his most eloquent, he was able to shed some light on how he experienced 'bad' things or conflict. Relating to the murder and his wife's violence, he remarked in an agitated way, 'bad is bad, that's it ... there is nothing else to it ... that is why I never think about it. It [badness] is there, paying attention to it never helped anyone.' He went on to say in the same session that he often found himself frustrated because he was never able to discipline his pupils or his own daughter for reasons unknown to him. He associated this with a fear that it would threaten the good relationships he maintained with them. He also made reference to how his wife's violence began to destroy the commitment he felt towards his pupils.

Grant reported having a number of female friends to whom he could relate, but never about his problems at home. Ironically they described him as 'problem free and happy-go-lucky'. During the court case the principal at his school testified that he was 'an exceptional and considerate teacher' who was responsible and hardworking. He also reported that Grant was non-aggressive in his manner and this made it difficult to believe that he could have committed murder.

Nothing out of the ordinary appears to have happened on the day of the murder, although his wife had continually argued with him the previous week. That night, whilst he was bathing his daughter, his wife began insulting him for not having done a particular chore. She then slapped him, throwing him into 'a different state of mind'. After this, she went to her room to say her daily prayers alone. At this point, filled with rage, Grant went to fetch his firearm and ran into her room shooting his wife several times whilst she was praying. Immediately following this, his daughter ran into the room and was also shot in the frenzy. These events were recalled with little emotion or insight and he disowned his actions completely when he spoke of his 'daughter's death':

> So after she slapped me I was in a sort of different state of mind ... I saw my drawer open, and my daughter – she had been standing there where the cupboard was. I can't remember much. I don't know, she [his daughter] was fiddling with some clothes or something like that, and I saw that open and I just went and grabbed the gun ... I think my wife had already gone to the other room ... I just ran in there and I just shot everywhere. Now in that state ... I never think about this, you know ... In some ways I have never really thought about it except now here with you ... Even before this thing [the murders], I never thought of doing this. On three occasions I remember wanting to hit her to teach her a lesson but I never ever did anything to her.

> So I think I remember turning around ... you know ... my hand was shaking because I saw blood and that coming out, you know ... she had been kneeling ... and I did turn around and I knocked my little girl, she had run into the room I think ... and then another shot went off and that shot hit her right on the head. That was a plain accident ... I don't know which angle or whatever it was, you know. That's all I remember.

On another occasion Grant claimed: 'I did not murder my daughter, she accidentally got in the way.' He talked about all this in a rather passive manner. The narrative reads as if the situation gives him a new opportunity to act differently. When he becomes active in committing the offence, it takes place whilst his wife is disengaged and passive. The gun had been purchased 3 years previously after Grant had been hijacked in his car. He had wanted to be able to defend himself in the event of it happening again.

As seen above, Grant admits to having had fantasies of hurting his wife, but never thought he was ever capable of extreme violence. Most dominant in his mind, however, were fears of being humiliated and attacked by others around him. He had no history of violent behaviour whatsoever.

The nature of the transference was clear from the outset and changed little throughout most of our time together. He was overly submissive and obliging. He found it difficult to speak freely and often wanted to make sure that he had given me the 'right' answer. Throughout the therapy there was also a clear sense of avoidance in talking about more difficult topics. He often changed the course of the session towards what was good and 'valuable' to him.

At one point he needed to leave the room during a particularly difficult session when he began to talk about an unbearable sense of shame he felt, something that he had worked hard to conceal from his mother. Attempts to contain the situation were fruitless at this point and he was unable to make use of interpretations that were aimed at encouraging him to think through what he felt to be unbearable. Just before the end of the session he returned but could not say anything more about what he felt. Towards the end of his therapy, however, Grant made some attempts to further elaborate on his sense of shame. He described a deep fear of 'being exposed to her [his mother] because her disappointment would stop her from loving [him]'.

There were also some indications of the transference changing when the crime or his wife's violent behaviour were alluded to. Initially, he 'forgot' to mention anything about his daughter in describing the crime. He was also careful to end his statements about his wife's violence by saying something 'good' about the difficult issues he was talking about. For example, he would follow talking about his wife's anger with overstated gestures about his need for her 'love and nurturance'.

Interestingly, in one of our sessions he kept on saying that he 'had left through the back door' to escape his wife's threats. After being questioned about this, however, he realized that the 'back door' reference had no literal relevance to what actually happened. Following some of his associations, I understood this to be an unconscious reference to his 'back door' way of coping with the abuse whereby he was able to shield himself from confronting the real implications of his conflictual relationship. A further significant slip occurred in his reference to his in-laws as '*late* in-laws'. In the context of the session it appeared most strongly associated with an unconscious attempt to make all things associated with his wife 'late' in his mind. I used these references to try and interpret his phobic responses to dealing with internal conflict. Through persistently interpreting his use of splitting and other defences associated with the 'narcissistic exoskeleton', he eventually displayed a greater capacity for reflection and grew to be more intrigued with his own thinking: a sign, I think, of some therapeutic progress when dealing with patients who show little interest in the creative capacities of their own internal worlds.

The most impressive feature of my countertransference was the depth of my empathy towards him. I felt sorry for Grant; I felt that he was essentially a good man who had suffered unduly. I found myself wanting to spend more time with him than I needed to. It was very difficult for me to believe that he had killed someone, particularly his own child, as he appeared to be the most unlikely perpetrator of such a crime. A further occurrence that appears significant in the transference–countertransference interaction occurred on a number of occasions when I found myself uncharacteristically finishing his sentences for him and sometimes talking over him.

My work with Grant supports the idea that a particular type of defensive organization renders rage-type offenders vulnerable to explosive violence. His most dominant object relations constellate around an idealized relationship with a maternal object that is easily transferred onto other situations. Here, the split between suffering vulnerable objects and more idealized parts of the personality are clear. The most stable identification apparent is characterized by passive submission in order to preserve or maintain a phantasy of ideal love and bliss. This part of him rejects all violence or associated themes, such as discipline, to ensure that his object remains in a symbiotic relationship with him. This pattern of relating is present in the transference–countertransference paradigm. His portrayal of a good, obliging person engenders a strong sense in me that he is not capable of an act such as the one he committed, as well as a sense of wanting to 'help' him by finishing his sentences. The above seems to represent a form of relating characterized by goodness and caring, with him in a passive state, very separate from the reality of the pain and difficulty that he had really been through.

I want to turn now to exploring the profile of some other intrapsychic dimensions of violence that are demonstrated by this case.

Representational capacity

As is the case with Grant, offenders who have committed rage offences show signs of an impoverished representational capacity. Often people are referred to in a concrete, one-dimensional fashion, with little acknowledgement of internal mental space. As discussed earlier in some detail, the inability to mentalize, manipulate and symbolize psychical processes leaves the individual more vulnerable to acts of violence. Mental objects remain concrete and are felt to be more associated with the body than with the mind, hence more prone to physical action. This sets up a curious position for rage offenders given that we have seen that they do not often have a history of violence – the 'fight' response. They would much rather take flight from conflict and aggression, internal or external. Their sophisticated defensive strategies appear to take care of that. It seems, however, that in such cases the flight response remains simply an action, a simple withdrawal, and seldom opens up representational space or gives the offender more room to think or process the event. As a result, threatening incidents are experienced as discrete encounters, having little mental life on which they could rely for more constructive ways of thinking. In Grant's case there are numerous references to him taking flight from conflict, eloping to get married, escaping his wife's abuse, needing to leave the therapy room. Although one might argue that these may have been 'constructive' responses given Grant's situation, it remains an escape, a simple action. The space created does not lead to further mentation, it is simply defensive.

TAT findings, collected from 22 rage offenders, 9 of whom had committed murder (Cartwright, 2000), further support my observations above. For my purpose I used a scoring system specifically designed by Westen (1991) to measure representational capacity and affect-tone (Barends et al., 1990). Briefly, it was clear here that the ability to discriminate between different objects was consistently poor. Also prominent were themes illustrating the inaccessibility of objects and the lack of exchange between them. Figures were represented as unidimensional in form. Much of the focus was on the actions of the object, with little attention being paid to the complexity of the character's internal world. There also existed a tendency to deny, or under-represent, conflictual or malevolent themes related to the self as identified in the cards. Furthermore, concrete cause–effect relationships typified their most prominent means of engagement with surroundings and there was little indication of thought-mediated action being present.

A poorly defined 'reflective self', to use Fonagy *et al.*'s (1993a) term, has a number of related implications. First, it delineates a relatively primitive psychological state where repression as a psychological defence cannot operate effectively. By definition, internalized objects or processes that are not 'mentalized' cannot be recognized as objects to be potentially repressed. By implication, the action of repression, a relatively mature defence, is unavailable to this part of the psyche. If one accepts this, it would be incorrect to conceptualize repression as the key reason to why aggression is mostly unexpressed until it eventually erupts or floods the psyche (when the repressive barrier ruptures). Further, if conflictual aspects of the self were adequately mentalized and subject to repression, a neurotic solution to rage would be much more available. Here symptom formation, sublimation, displacement and other neurotic mechanisms would at least deal with some of the repressed affect–idea constellation.

Second, without an adequate capacity to *re*-present one's own emotional states to oneself, the ability to 'think about' and work through psychic pain is foreclosed. The suffering of self and others cannot be truly acknowledged or tolerated which, in turn, makes the process of mourning and psychic digestion a formidable task. This is apparent in a number of different ways in the cases I have explored; I shall only mention the most prominent.

In Grant's case his wife's persistent abuse cannot be 'thought about' in a way that gives him some 'psychological distance' from its traumatic effects. As a result, his experience of a 'traumatic' incident is equated with the incident itself. Similarly, Simon, the reader may recall, often spoke about his past abusive relationship in the present tense as if the trauma continually occurred inside him. This, in my view, was a clear indication of how Simon managed past traumatic experience; it remained concrete, immovable and ever present, and in so doing stood in the way of his ability to mourn. This kind of impasse, however, does not only occur as a result of past traumatic experience. I have suggested that the internal situation observed in such individuals is perpetuated by a particular defensive style. Earlier, in reviewing current work in this area, it was also argued that more subtle interactional styles may also have an impact on representational capacity. Still further, as we shall see later, it appears that factors related to overstimulation, idealizing interactional patterns and symbiotic relations may in themselves adequately account for the retardation of the 'reflective self'.

It has to be said, however, that poor representational capacity should be understood not only within the context of a predisposed personality. It may also be influenced by contemporary stressors that lead to the collapse of the 'reflective self', in turn, shortening the pathway to action even more. Certainly, particularly in Ralph's case, the trauma of his brother's death is clearly a key factor to be considered in understanding a collapse into more concrete forms of thought. 'My kind of manner changed after my brother [had died]', he said once, 'I would kind of think in pictures, like I would see my brother lying dead, or just see images of my family, but I couldn't really talk to myself about it'. Ralph's description appears to make reference to his return to ideographic forms of thought (Bion, 1962b) where psychic digestion is eluded and transformation into representational thought fails.

In general, offenders make reference to an inability to *re*-present their own aggressive potential. Often they indicate that if they had 'known' about their own aggression they would have had a better chance of avoiding the final outburst. Grant made reference to this a number of times in claiming that if he had been able to talk about his aggression to his mother she would have been able to help him. Similarly, Ralph claims, 'I was a mediator of conflict, helping others. If I had known I could get that bad, maybe I would have thought about it first instead of losing it ... I had nothing to measure that by.'

A third implication, following on from Fonagy and his colleagues' understanding of the 'reflective self', relates to the importance of representational capacity in creating mental space. The retardation of this process has implications for the individual's sense of psychological space, feelings of entrapment, claustrophobic phenomena and so forth. This kind of experience has often been noted in borderline dynamics (Meltzer, 1992; Rey, 1988; Steiner, 1993). On reviewing the buildup to the murder in some of the cases, a lack of mental space may well have contributed to a claustrophobic sense of feeling consumed by the situation. The experience is felt to be endless and annihilatory and must therefore be stopped through violence.

All the above go some way in explaining the offenders' inability to 'think through' their problematic situations or the distress they were experiencing at the time of the murder. This often makes psychotherapy very difficult and places specific demands on the therapist. Here, thinking in the presence of another is felt to be extremely painful. A patient of mine, who experienced similar problems, once aptly likened this process to having to 'slave-drive' his mind 'in order to get it working'. Clearly, for him, thinking was an arduous and exhausting process that he felt often led to nothing fruitful. I shall say a little more about the problems this causes in treating such offenders in the final chapter.

Although rage offenders tend to display problems with representational capacity, this does not appear to be invariable across situations. In other words, they do not display a blanket incapacity to represent their internal worlds. If that were so, one would expect these offenders to have a history of impulsive behaviour along with intermittent explosive episodes. There are two other factors associated with other intrapsychic dimensions that help explain this. The first relates to the defensive organization discussed earlier; the second relates to external situational factors.

Referring to the former, representational capacity appears to differ across the split between the idealized self-object system and the bad-object system. The representational capabilities of the idealized system appears to be far greater than those of the bad encapsulated self. Grant, for example, spent a great deal of time explaining the 'pleasures' in his life to me and what he thought they stood for. Included in these ruminations where his thoughts of how his wife loved him, his adoration for his mother and the nature of his somewhat compulsive religious convictions. He did this in relatively elaborate and sophisticated ways. When asked to reflect on his own emotional state, however, he had great difficulty. As alluded to earlier, he also struggled considerably when I tried to encourage him to think about more conflictual and contradictory parts of his life.

Some of the details related to the nature of representational problems were apparent in offenders' responses to the Rorschach.[1] Notably, the average response rate, in a group of 22 offenders, was particularly low (an average of 13 responses) and responses in the inquiry phase were often very brief and lacked elaboration. Form level was also generally poor. This was particularly the case when responses were negative or displayed aggressive content. This appeared to support the idea that poorer representational capacity could be associated with the bad-object system. Although the poor response rate and the quality of responses posed some problems for assessing object relations in detail, these findings in themselves indicated the high level of defensiveness apparent in such offenders as well as the impoverished nature of their internal worlds. The general inability to use fantasy to elaborate on the cards also appears to reflect an impoverished ability to make use of 'potential space' in the Winnicottian sense of the word (Smith, 1990). Here, reality – in this case, the 'reality' of the card as an inkblot – is used as a defence against fantasy. As Smith suggests, these kind of responses are often recorded in patients who appear 'quite normal on the surface' (p.789). As we have seen in exploring the defensive organization, 'normality' essentially amounts to acts of defensive compliance where reality and the external world are clung to in a defensive attempt to ward off the bad-object system.

There were minimal signs of aggressive content or aggressive potential in Rorschach responses, whilst chromatic colour and shading determinants were prominent relative to other determinants. This finding is in keeping with Meloy and Gacono's (1992) assertion that this is typical of individuals who are capable of affective forms of violence. Notably, in an ideographic analysis of some of the cases, when there were aggressive responses recorded, such responses often displayed a particular kind of defensiveness and initial responses were sometimes rejected for more acceptable options. For example, Grant's response to card two was as follows: 'There are two creatures facing each other. They were fighting and

---

1 Rorschach protocols were scored using Exner's (1986) Comprehensive System. In addition, Blatt *et al.*'s (1976) differentiation scale as well as Meloy and Gacono's (1992) proposed aggressive indices were used to assess the quality of object relations and the nature of the aggressive response.

hurting each other. No, sorry, they were playing, playing not fighting. The one wants to get inside that whole.' On inquiry, the aggressive response was initially determined by the colour in the card. These kinds of response appear to illustrate a defensive style typified by an overcontrolling reaction that is used to manage, or cover up, anything that approximates aggressive 'bad' experience, in turn, not allowing any mental elaboration of this part of the self.

More generally, it follows that given that this part of the psyche, the 'bad self', is not perceived as consciously being part of the self, it would comprise less mental space than other areas. This implies that the vulnerability to act violently is not only precipitated by the sensitivity and exposure of split-off bad objects when narcissistic defences break down; it also has its roots in a deficiency in the ability to mentalize. But how should we formulate the origins of violence when considering the representational capacity of these offenders?

It could be that aggressiveness serves as a means of defending an already fickle psychological self, as Fonagy *et al.* (1991) have it. On the other hand, the key aggressive dynamic could be the opposite where it serves to attack the representational self and the ability to think (Bion, 1970; Fonagy *et al.*, 1993b; Segal, 1978). It appears that the narcissistic defensive structure found in these offenders works in this way to prevent the creation of new thoughts and the elaboration of the internal world. Whether poor representational capacity is a consequence of defensiveness or the result of a deficit in the personality is a very difficult question to answer and still requires further investigation. Put another way, does poor representational capacity occur due to the 'shielding' function of the narcissistic exoskeleton, or is it more the result of chronic and direct damage to the self. Clearly, this is an important question to explore given its implications for clinical work and the prognosis of such offenders. It is not enough, I believe, simply to assume that poor representational capacity stems from deficits in the personality because rage offenders generally fit an atypical borderline profile. One could argue that these individuals show few signs that would otherwise indicate severe deficits in ego functioning. I am referring here to signs of psychosis, chronic instability, or emotional lability. But the kind of stability and pseudo-digestive capabilities evident as a consequence of the 'narcissistic exoskeleton' diminishes this claim. Although not conclusive, my therapeutic work with rage offenders – not necessarily murderers – suggests that, in time, when defences are addressed, representational capacity does improve. I have indicated that this was evident in my work with Grant. The point made earlier about representational capacity being variable also lends some support to the argument that defensive style plays an important role here.

The nature and quality of the object world

Apart from representational capacity, there are a number of other factors of significance in the nature of the offender's internal world. With no history of violence prior to the murder, the 'target selection', to use Meloy's (1988) term, of these offenders appears to be very narrow and finite. Following Meloy, one of the implications of this is that offenders of this type are unlikely to commit murder again. Although this is difficult to prove, given that offenders are imprisoned for long periods of time and 'prevented' from re-offence, some have found support for this claim (Blackburn, 1993; Carney 1974; Meloy, 1992).

Although internalized objects are poorly represented in the psyche, offenders are still able to select particular objects as targets of violence. Grant's wife was clearly a key figure in his 'split' object world. She represents the precarious, but well-defended tension between his idealizing capabilities and his disowned aggression. She, I would argue, was carefully selected as a life partner, and cannot be separated from, for this reason. Once this tension collapses, however, she is destined to be a target. Ralph, to use another example, did not attack just anyone during his catathymic turmoil. He killed his ex-girlfriend because she was equated with bad festering elements of the self that were controlled at a distance. She had become the initial threatening object that breached his narcissistic defences, forcing him to confront the 'deadly force', to use his words, that lay within him. The act of rage as it is experienced here is far from being 'objectless' in nature. Even at moments when explosive affect is in ascendance, the offender's rage is clearly directed by internal object relations in which the victim plays a part.

This in itself, however, is not an adequate explanation for the actions leading to murder. Grant clearly had felt threatened in other situations that did not lead to the expression of murderous rage towards his wife. As is being argued here, a number of dimensions ultimately contribute to the act. But the nature of most of the relationships observed between murderer and victim may further help understand the role the target object plays in the offender's mind. There are two factors to be considered here that are illustrated in Grant's case. First, often an internalized threat, associated in some way with the target object, is sustained and experienced over a long period of time. The full repercussions of this insidious process is continually denied. The net effect is a build-up of considerable resentment that remains largely unconscious.

The second observation relates to the fact that relationships with the victim are usually close or intimate in nature. This tends to set up an entrapping dynamic as the closeness of this relationship also means that the victim becomes the ultimate ally in supporting the offender's defensive strategies. As we have seen earlier, the victim-to-be is often the main object tightly embroiled in the offender's narcissistic defences. At this level, the trigger event is felt to be the ultimate act of betrayal. Once this occurs, bad aspects of the object/victim are experienced as being forced into the offender whilst he is vulnerable and defenceless.

What can we discern from this regarding a general capacity for object relating? As mentioned earlier, rage offenders are often reasonably successful and live relatively normal lives. This suggests that some nourishing engagement with external objects must have taken place. Although this is an important factor regarding the relative stability of the individual, my observations suggest that object relations have a narcissistic core. Rage offenders lack the capacity to relate to an object's interior and are only able to see the object as a reflection of self. Relating is thus flat, unemotional and removed. In this way objects are somewhat dehumanized and devoid of realistic qualities. Although close relationships are ostensibly important to these men, these key figures are seldom portrayed by the offender as having their own thoughts and feelings. Objects are most often portrayed in a idealistic way, another means of maintaining distance from the realistic qualities and demands, good and bad, of the object.

I have suggested earlier that 'imitation', as a primitive precursor to identification, may help us further understand the nature of object relations that make up the offender's internal world. Essentially, imitation refers to a primitive identification process whereby behaviours are appropriated through imitation of the object. The objects, however, are not internalized and thus depend on the constant presence of the external object. Over-compliance, a key defensive pattern in rage offenders, seems to have its source in a constant imitation of what is perceived to be 'good', as opposed to a process where an individual draws upon his own internal resources to inform his own behaviour. The idea that imitation occurs at this level is also supported by there being few signs of an adequately internalized sense of 'goodness' in the individuals I have worked with. That they have not internalized 'a sense of goodness', on the face of it, appears to be a relatively predictable statement to make about most criminals. But what is intriguing about these offenders is their ability to simulate 'a sense of goodness' in a way that is deceptive to themselves and others. Usually this leaves its mark in the minds of others, who, after the murder, spend a great deal of time trying to reconcile the dissonance between their murderous actions and their often much admired outward personas.

References to maternal objects appear to vary somewhat. In a majority of the cases, however, maternal objects are represented in an idealized way, associated with a theme of over-protection and dependence. As alluded to earlier, this has been noted by a number of authors. One of the cornerstones of Meloy's (1992) argument, for instance, is that pathological attachments with the primary object emerge again in the build-up to the murder. Weiss *et al.* (1960), on the other hand, focused on the entrapping qualities that surround the maternal object. Here, dependence on the all-good loving mother leads to the repression of inevitable hostility that arises as a consequence of over-protectiveness.

Importantly, in my own analysis, references to the maternal object are consistently linked to the emergence of the 'narcissistic exoskeleton'. A mutual over-protective and idealizing form of relating between offender and maternal object, so characteristic of the defensive system observed here, appears to explain partly how the 'narcissistic exoskeleton' is established. Here, concern for the primary object, or a transference figure, is first and foremost aimed at ensuring that affirmation and idealization are reflected back from the object in order to uphold the 'good' self.

It is possible that Brenman Pick's (1995) observations regarding excessive concern for an object may be relevant here. She discusses a group of patients who display a spurious kind of concern which predates more genuine forms of concern that belong to the depressive position. In her analysis of two patients she finds that the pivotal dynamic that lies behind such apparent concern involves the manic 'take over' of the maternal function. In her words: 'there is an early "take over" of the breast, in which the infant "becomes" the breast and shows behaviour which is in part a fake of a very concerned mother' (p.257). The manoeuvre is primarily an attempt to overcompensate for deprivation experienced and to avoid negotiating the painful demands of separateness. Like other offenders, Grant's often overstated statements of caring, being concerned, and wanting to constantly 'do for others', appears closely to resemble Brenman Pick's descriptions.

Viewing the idealized maternal object as being embroiled in the creation of the defensive system certainly appears to resonate with Shengold's (1991) main contention about rage reactions and murder. Overstimulation, according to him, creates an idealized system of object relations that are believed to resemble the true self. When this collapses it is not only experienced as an annihilation of the self, but also brings with it the sense of being betrayed or deceived by the original maternal object. This appears to have been part of the repetition that Grant played out with his wife where she, as the part-idealized object, constantly betrayed this belief. But he has an over-determined investment in this image of her and constantly reinvolves himself in ways that attempt to comply with her and win her back. In some cases the fear of idealized objects abandoning or deceiving the offender evokes a paralysing sense of shame where the threat of separation exposes extreme inadequacy. Grant sometimes associated this with a fear of 'losing his mind'; a fear which I think was paralleled by a phantasy of 'losing himself' if his narcissistic defences collapsed.

As discussed earlier, attachment formations with the primary object have implications for understanding violent behaviour (Bowlby, 1969; Zulueta, 1993). From an object-relations perspective, however, it is not the attachment *per se* that explains the offender's murderous actions. We need to understand the implications attachment problems have for the internal object world. Certainly, there is often a history of attachment and separation difficulties in such cases. Therefore I would agree with Meloy, Zulueta and others that attachment – predominantly anxious attachment – is a key issue here. Our investigation, thus far, seems to say more about what lies behind this attachment pattern. In my experience separation is felt to be traumatic principally because the primary object has become the repository for the offender's 'good' self, a crucial aspect of their defensive organization. Separation from the object thus not only feels like a loss of the self in a very concrete way; it further means the loss of an essential means of defending the self. In other words, in times of threat, the other – originally the maternal object – is desperately needed to *close* and maintain the psychological system.

The absence of a constant, supportive paternal object has been a remarkably consistent finding across cases I have explored. The internal representations of the paternal object are poorly developed and they are felt to be inaccessible or rejecting. The general implications of this have already been outlined in some detail regarding how this affects the individual's self-reflective and symbolic capacities. Without a third object there is no point of reference outside symbiotic object relations, adding to a sense of entrapment that may already have been felt to come from the maternal object. Despite an escalating conflictual situation, Grant felt a third object to be inaccessible and thus did not seek help or intervention. 'For some reason,' he said to me once, 'I did not think of outside help. Nobody knew, there was nobody between us. I've always felt it good to keep it between me and the other person ... or just keep it to myself.' In some cases I have explored, help from a third party was sought during times of conflict, but this did not seem to modify the escalating situation in any way.

The absence of a significant third object is also supported, to some extent, by a consideration of the precipitant emotions that exist just prior to the murder. If the internal drama being played out here included a third object, we would expect the motives for the murders to be overshadowed by themes of revenge, jealousy and sexual conflict. This, however, is not the case. Certainly, infidelity, rejection and the denial of the real implications of such problems may play an important role in the escalation of conflict. But, as we have seen, the representational space neces- sary to think about such conflicts appears to be limited, prompting a regression to a position where the object is experienced as concrete and one-dimensional. For this reason it appears more accurate to conceptualize violent action as emerging from a more primitive object constellation motivated by annhilatory fear.

In some cases signs of conflict between son and father, self and paternal object are apparent, but aggression is constantly denied or cannot be expressed. In Andrew's case, for instance, anger towards his father could only be acknowledged after the murder, in turn enabling him to mourn what was previously split off. Prior to this, all elements associated with aggression, good or bad, are internalized as part of a defensive manoeuvre, still remaining dissociated in the psyche. Similarly, Simon recalled being aware of his anger towards his father in some instances. He could never express this, however, and on occasions when he did have contact with his father, he was left with a sense of helplessness and sometimes had thoughts of suicide that he could not explain. It appears that his observations here illustrate his usual coping style where anger and its toxic and dangerous associations are re-internalized and turned on the self as a means of protection.

Significantly, identifications with male figures are always somewhat precarious, adding to a more vulnerable position regarding challenges to the offender's masculinity. We shall discuss this further in considering the role of sexuality. In terms of precarious identifications *per se,* Perelberg (1995a) has noted, in her detailed analysis of a number of violent patients, how rapid oscillations between male and female identifications contribute to a violent outcome. Here, female identifications are experienced as extremely threatening, initiating violent out- bursts. Along with the nature of the primary object relationship discussed above and the absence of the paternal object, entrapping female identifications play an important role in predisposing offenders to extreme violence. This appears to be the underside of the idealization of the maternal relationship: a deeply hidden, shameful experience, of feeling more like the mother whilst having little access to a paternal object.

The quality of the superego does not always appear to be excessively aggressive or destructive in the case of the rage-type murderer. With that having been said, this is often difficult to assess given the submissive and appeasing nature of the ego or representations of self that, at first glance, obscure any trace of conflict. However, the superego does have other salient qualities. The split between 'internal' and 'external'[2] objects, consistent with the defensive organization, gives the superego a 'Janus-faced' or 'two-faced quality'. Towards external objects it is allied with the compliant ego, moulding itself to gain complementarity with the object in order to ensure that no confrontation or conflict occurs.

On the other hand, when the superego is turned inward, whilst still allied with the defensive system, it attacks damaged internalized objects due to their association with 'badness'. The 'Janus-faced' nature of the superego appears to account for the overly righteous and moralistic attitude evident in most rage offenders further contributing to the rigidity of the defensive system. Their righteous attitude would read as follows if it could be stated outright: 'I will not only keep the external world free from destruction, damage and badness. I will take it all into myself and destroy it.' For this to be effective the real implications of damage are denied. As mentioned earlier, damaged internalized objects are obscured by their strong association with the split-off bad-object system. Here, damage to the self is shameful and equated with 'badness'. As a result internal resources that might otherwise have been capable of containing or supporting parts of the self that had suffered in some way cannot be used. Most of the time, as we have seen with Grant, this attitude is epitomized by disdain for recognizing one's own suffering.

As mentioned earlier, Glasser's (1978) division of the superego into proscriptive and prescriptive aspects provides a useful means of thinking about the 'Janus-faced' nature of the superego in these offenders. To recapitulate, the *proscribed superego* is concerned with moral restrictions and prohibitions. The *prescribed superego*, on the other hand, functions to set goals and ideals as well as ways of attaining them. Applied to rage-type offenders, the proscribed superego has a harsh restrictive quality that is largely turned in on the self. The prescriptive superego, on the other hand, 'abandons' internal objects and bases all goals and affirmations on interactions with external objects. When this fails, the individual is exposed to feelings of shame and worthlessness. Most important here, however, is the split that occurs between 'internal'/'external' and the proscribed/prescribed superego. This often emerges in contradictory attitudes offenders have, particularly towards situations that depict some kind of suffering. At one point, Grant had this

---

2 'External' is not used here to refer to actual external objects. I use the word 'external' and 'internal' here to depict how internal objects are organized in the individual's phantasies. Here, the split between what is shown to the external world depicts 'external' objects and what is shielded from view depicts the 'internal' bad self.

to say about other's suffering: 'People are hurt easily you know. But this is easily sorted out, I have helped many people like this. If you treat them well you feel well. I'm sure that's why you like your job as a shrink?' Disguised behind this apparent benevolence we find the prescribed superego's attempts to set out the basis for interaction with others where the goal is to create a façade of idealism. When Grant tries to talk about his own suffering, however, his ideas are quite different. In the same session as the above quote he claims that he has never thought he had really needed help because, in his words, 'I somehow don't get hurt, suffering is weak ... I keep to myself and move on.' This statement seems to reflect the kind of prohibitions he places on himself, particularly related to suffering.

It appears that the conflation of 'damage' and 'badness' possibly also serves to vindicate the offender from overwhelming feelings of guilt related to the destruction of damaged objects. For this reason it seems unlikely that attacks are motivated by a persecutory sense of guilt found by Anderson (1997) to be an important factor in attacks on damaged objects. Here, attacking an already damaged object serves to annihilate any traces of guilt related to the original damage done. Possibly, this dynamic holds some meaning when a 'second attack' follows the initial murderous outburst. In this case the damage already done in the first instance is obliterated, in phantasy, in the second attack. Although Grant denies almost all responsibility for killing his daughter, the way he describes the incident suggests it may have occurred as a result of the above dynamic. As we have seen, it is also 'forgotten' in his recalling of events to me perhaps as a means of committing a similar internal action where unbearable thoughts that identify him as an aggressive murderer are eliminated from his mind.

Interaction with the external situation

On reviewing the importance of the external situation as an intrapsychic dimension of violence, I pointed out that the crime scene, and the events leading up to the crime, allow another point of access into understanding the internal word of the violent offender. A number of these factors have already been mentioned such as provocation, absence of a plan and the 'overkill' nature of the murder. Indicators like these tell us about the explosive mental state of the offender at the time of the murder. In the build-up to the crime, the nature of the relationship between victim and murderer also reflects certain aspects of the offender's psychological make-up. In most cases the offender's behaviour and thought associations point to some dependence on the victim. If this is the case, one wonders how much of the conscious sense of entrapment felt by some of the offenders is not also the reflection of an unconscious need for the object, no matter how problematic it is in reality. The general inability to play an assertive or constructive role in interaction with others appears to serve a simple but important purpose: to avoid any confrontation of the defensive splitting that has occurred in the personality. Furthermore, the offender puts himself in a position where he need not take any responsibility for inevitable conflict or difficulty. Although a relatively benign position to adopt, its effects are insidious and catastrophic. Unaware of the implications of this, the offender slowly pushes himself into a desperate and helpless position where the only means of escape is defensive attack.

Most often offenders find themselves immersed in problematic situations in the build-up to the murder. This undoubtedly impacts on their internal world rendering them more vulnerable, fragile and consequently more defensive. Grant, for instance, had been subjected to considerable abuse from his wife leading to two divorces, whilst Ralph was trying to deal with the daunting news that his brother had been killed. But to what extent do factors such as these drive an individual to murder? Would anyone under these kinds of stressor commit murder? Of course, this would not be the case. These factors would have certainly contributed to these individuals' vulnerability, but they cannot explain why particular intrapsychic pathways or processes occur in one individual and not another.

There are often specific features of the interaction prior to the murder that appear to further contribute to the offender's actions. It has already been argued that particular dissociative processes in the psyche predispose them to rage. But there is another way of understanding dissociative statements such as 'the anger did not feel like a part of me', as Grant put it. Such statements might easily be understood as being part of their experience of dissociation consistent with the split in the personality. From an interactional perspective, however, statements like this may have a more literal interpretation. It is possible that murderousness or unmanageable experience is not felt to be a part of them because it belongs to their victim, but is forced into them via projective identification. In other words, the offender becomes an unwilling recipient of the victim's projections. Of course, parts of the self are not magically transferred from one person to the other. The phantasy of evacuation, conveyed via projective identification, is realized in interaction with the other, where the manipulation of the interpersonal field prompts the desired response. In other words, the individual unconsciously 'prods' his recipient so that he responds in a way that confirms that he has unburdened himself of toxic internal objects. Hyatt-Williams (1998) describes a similar interaction whereby both parties juggle an indigestible projection. An escalating conflictual situation ensues that can no longer be tolerated by the offender who then, after re-projecting the intolerable experience, attacks it in the victim. We established earlier that in threatening situations the offender already battles to contain his own aggressive or 'bad' propensities. If one adds to this the threat of intrusive projections from others, forcing him to have contact with split-off aspects of himself, the individual is bound to be more vulnerable to defensive attack. This scenario is best observed in cases where the victims themselves are reported to have been violent. This possibility presents itself when we reconstruct Grant's situation just prior to his explosive attack. It is possible here that the final violent provocation is felt to be an intrusive projection from his wife, forcing an identification with evacuated dangerous parts of the self. It cannot be contained and is returned with even greater force and aggression. Likewise, one might infer that Andrew experienced his partner's aggressive threats as indigestible and therefore dangerous. If one accepts this, his only defence was to return the intrusive projections and annihilate them in his victim.

Viewed from this perspective, if taken to its extreme, the victims themselves play a crucial role in their own murder. They become the original perpetrators of violent action whilst the offenders become the vulnerable recipients who can no longer contain what is projected into them. In essence, it is the offender who is the victim here. This should not be taken to mean that the offender is exonerated from responsibility for the crime in any way, as some perpetrators may sometimes claim. The offender's intrapsychic make-up, particularly their defensive organization, still holds the key to why such an interaction ends in murder. It is also unlikely that the interactional sequence is ever as clear as outlined above. In an escalating violent situation the boundaries between self and other become far less distinguishable along with the constructs of 'victim' and 'offender', projector and recipient. One might argue that such situations are more about a 'borderline situation' than they are about a borderline personality. Here, the confusion between self and object is constituted *between* the individuals in the interaction. Often, the aftermath of such crimes are shrouded in a sense of tragedy. In some ways, the tragedy expressed here portrays an accurate sense that the murderous impulse cannot simply be located in either one of the parties. Even more, it conveys a sense that the situation was less about cold-blooded murder and more about unbearable distress.

Chapter 8

Trauma, phantasy/fantasy and sexuality

I turn now to exploring the last three dimensions of rage-type murder. I shall argue that past traumatic experience, although significant in some cases, is not a necessary condition for violence. How the effects of trauma are internalized appears to be a more important question to ask here. We shall also see that contemporary stress or trauma appears to be a more significant triggering factor in this kind of violence. Earlier, I put forward the idea that the phantasy/fantasy distinction provides a useful means of exploring different forms of violence. In explosive violence phantasies of engulfment and compensatory idealization appear most evident. Significant too is the relative absence of murderous conscious fantasy in many such cases.

In considering the final dimension, some thoughts about sexuality and sexualization, and how they relate to explosive violence, will be explored. I have chosen a case that appears clearly to illustrate the role of the above dimensions in such offenders. This particular individual, whom I shall call Ben, endured a long period of sexual abuse that had traceable implications throughout his life. Here, the 'narcissistic exoskeleton' predominantly finds its roots in sexual expression of a very particular kind.

BEN

Ben, a 32-year-old man, killed his girlfriend, Jane, by stabbing her 15 times in a blind rage whilst she lay sleeping in her bed. They had just got back together again after a 2-month separation.

Ben grew up in a modest home. His father was a construction supervisor, and his mother a housewife. He had an older brother and sister, and one younger brother. Both his parents appeared to be very ineffectual. His mother was an alcoholic and spent most of the time preoccupied with her own problems. His father simply took very little interest in the family. As a result, Ben spent most of his time at his uncle's house just down the road. From ages 5–16 Ben reported that he was consistently sexually abused by his uncle without any intervention from others around him. The abuse took place within the context of a seductive relationship in which he was given toy cars and other gifts in return for sexual favours. He had this to say about their relationship:

> It went on for a long time and although my uncle did that [sexually abuse him] to me, and I did it, even when I was older, he cared for me greatly and gave me nice things ... he cared for me greatly. He would care about school and ask me how things were going and protect me from being bullied. He was a parent. I know it was wrong ... When I moved away, I never thought back about it. It was wrong but I never hated him or anything like that, he helped.

Although never directly associated with his uncle, he saw most men as being 'spineless' and weak, but at the same time, extremely threatening. He reacted by avoiding relating to men in any meaningful way. At times, Ben also made reference to himself as also feeling 'spineless' in the presence of women. He felt that he had been left feeling 'transparent' and all women could see the 'horrible things he had been up to'. He also felt that this was the reason why women had left him in the past, although he had never mentioned the abuse to anyone.

It was striking how, despite inquiry, his parents were virtually non-existent in his thoughts. When he was pushed to think about them, there were few indications of any negative or positive affective attachments towards them.

Ben found it very difficult to break away from his abusive relationship with his uncle. It was only once he had found a girlfriend, at age 16, that he became able to resist the pattern of 'abuse and reward' that characterized the relationship. Following school, at age 18, he left home to undergo his compulsory military training. Reports indicate that he refused to carry a gun and took up special 'pacifist' duties in his unit. As he puts it, 'I would rather be shy and keep to myself than be a loud aggressive person. I hate aggressive types who want to solve stuff through violence'. Such statements, of course, tended to contradict his own violent actions. Ben was never able to identify his own capacity for violence when talking about the violence of others.

After the army he began working in the construction trade and managed to earn a reasonable living. He had a number of brief sexual encounters but was unable to sustain a relationship. Eventually he married a woman he had met at work whom he described as being extremely withdrawn and passive. The relationship only lasted 2 years, however, after which she broke it off. From what I could establish, it appears that the most significant factor leading to the break-up was his excessive demands for sex. Still, Ben was puzzled about why she had left and could not understand why their sexual relationship was a problem.

He spoke of his wife as being 'the only woman I could love even though she was very shy and kept to herself'. Interestingly, his usual associations regarding his own passivity and shameful feelings disappeared when he talked about the details of his relationship with his wife. He felt 'comfortable', unthreatened and in control with her. He also made a number of references to feeling the same way in relating to adolescent or young children. This stood in stark contrast to his descriptions of feeling threatened in the presence of adult figures.

A year after his divorce he met Jane, a highly paid businesswoman with whom he had an intimate relationship for 7 months. Their relationship was characterized by excess. Jane spent large amounts of money on Ben, often buying him extravagant gifts and giving him 'extra money' on a weekly basis. They had a very active and experimental sexual relationship, with Jane often wanting him to perform sexual acts that he was not always comfortable with.

Almost all of Ben's relationships, before and after his marriage, seemed to be an arena for the expression of excessive sexual demands. 'When I found a woman who wanted sex the way I did', he recalled, 'I somehow felt we could relate on the same level.' But these relationships were also associated with the 'dirty feelings' that he felt had come from his relationship with his uncle. He said once, 'I feel dirty sometimes, but I carry on because I know that is what others want. I enjoy, but its dirty. I suppose I served Jane like I did with my uncle.' As expressed here, despite his haunting feelings related to sex, he finds himself preoccupied with thoughts of being able to satisfy other women and he would often go to extremes to achieve this.

> I would spend hours sometimes playing with them until I knew they were satisfied, whatever they wanted. In return, they kind of loved me. I'm not being great or anything, but I think I have a special power with females. They would come back for more ... If they didn't [come back] I would be angry but I just left it, I wouldn't say anything.

As Ben begins to indicate here women appeared to become a lot more threatening to him when his 'satisfying' fantasy could not be realized. He reported a brief dream that appears to illustrate this theme well. In his words, ' I was fucking Jane. She was loving it in a kind of admiring way ... but then the dream changed and she's not doing anything, like she stops digging it, and then she turns into this weird evil-devil-thing.'

The dream appeared to express a salient theme that also appeared to be prominent in his interactions with significant others: Jane is being satisfied sexually by him, but as soon as there are no signs of this being achieved, she turns into an 'evil-devil-thing'. Potential female objects of hate also emerge in his references to a separation from another girlfriend where he took to cutting up and destroying some of her belongings once she was gone. Here, perhaps are some of the more subtle signs of his aggressive potential and his propensity to murder, something he never imagined he was capable of.

Two months prior to the murder, Jane had called their relationship off for no specified reason. She also wanted him to return some of the belongings that she had bought him, most notably the new motorcycle she had purchased for him. He refused and it was left at that. Ben reports that after this they had no contact with each other until the day before the murder. That night they bumped into each other and decided to try to talk about why they had separated. After making up and deciding to continue their relationship they spent a night of heavy drinking on the town.

They returned to her flat where they began to have sex. At this point he remembered feeling frustrated because he was unable to maintain his erection, preventing them from continuing. He also recalled her falling off to sleep after sex was interrupted. It is difficult to know precisely what happened next, but shortly after this it appears that he too must have fallen asleep. In the morning he awoke and, although he could not recall this, he must have gone to the kitchen, got a bread knife, and returned to kill her. The court report indicates that he must have stood over her whilst she was sleeping and, in a fit of inexplicable rage, continually stabbed her. Ben eventually gave himself up to the police a few days later.

In talking to Ben, I was struck by the way he spoke about Jane. His statements left me with a sense that, in some unrealistic way, he felt she was still alive. The closest he came to conveying this verbally emerged in our last session:

> This is silly but sometimes I feel like I never did it, even now. All evidence points to me and I remember seeing her in blood you know ... the knife and stuff. But I feel that someone else may have come in and did it ... Although I feel bad about what I have done, I feel when I look at others that I cannot feel sorrow about the whole thing because it's like it didn't happen.

There were two prominent narrative themes associated with the attack. First, he and his girlfriend had separated and she had tried to take gifts from him that she had given him. He claimed that the separation meant nothing to him emotionally. Associations in other parts of the interviews, however, suggest that separations had led to hateful aggressive reactions in the past. Second, his inability to fulfil Jane's sexual needs clearly frustrated him that night and appears to be linked to a fear that he would no longer be able to satisfy women.

At no time in Ben's history had he been violent towards anyone. This was corroborated by a number of the witnesses at his trial. He claimed that he had not experienced any homicidal or aggressive thoughts prior to the murder. He had, however, felt some anger towards Jane regarding her attempts to take some of his 'gifts' away.

Throughout my interviews with Ben he was very softly spoken, reserved and avoided eye contact for much of the time. Often I felt he needed to avoid any real contact with me and on two occasions made reference to feeling intimidated by me. A large part of the interview time was taken up by him talking about his relationships with three significant women in his life. Significantly, he continuously confused one with the other. He also often distinctively referred to them as 'these females', leaving me with a sense of him not referring to them as if they were 'real people'. Apart from references to his uncle, men were hardly mentioned. There were some references in the interviews related to feeling trapped and badly treated by men. There were also many references to him feeling that only 'females' were able to understand him.

The most dominant feelings and thoughts impressed on me during the interviews related to a sense of 'unreality' whilst trying to listen to his story. Similarly, thoughts Ben had about his own future goals were markedly unrealistic and idealistic, although not psychotic. For instance, his main goal was to buy a large yacht and sail the world, something that was highly unlikely given his life situation. He showed little acknowledgement that possible achievements would have to take place in a world where there would be realistic limitations, where others' thoughts and feelings needed to be considered. This appears to be in stark contrast to his apparent sensitivity towards others, especially concerning sexual needs, where he sees himself as a 'servant' to others.

Reflecting on the above observations, what can be said about Ben's internal world? Indeed, supportive parental references or objects are conspicuous by their absence in Ben's narratives. The central object constellation centres around internalizations and identifications that emanate from his protracted abusive relationship with his uncle.

The primary object here is no longer his mother. Ben's uncle dominates object relations, forming a perverse symbiotic relationship with him. Here, the primary object appears to be split in two. On the one hand, he is perceived as being a seductive 'caring' figure, on the other, he is an extremely threatening, evil and powerful figure. Although the latter is not consciously acknowledged, his distorted perception of male figures suggests an underlying threat that has been disowned. Standing opposite this internal object, Ben identifies predominantly with a weak, timid, needy, childlike figure.

The threatening part of this object remains associated with men and is, in part, split off, but still prevents any meaningful contact with men. This was evident in the initial transference impressions that emerged in the interview as well as in the numerous references made about him struggling with relating to male adult figures. Consistent with his attempts to disown the real impact of the abuse, the seductive–gratifying object relationship is displaced and actualized in his relationships with women. Representations of the 'female' object are complex. For him, they provide a primitive form of gratification for the desperate needy part of him, conveyed mainly through sex and excessive gift giving. But the same objects also allow for a reversal of this object relationship where he is able to act out the role of the 'seductive gratifier', inducing in him a sense of omnipotence. All this appears closely related to re-enactments of his abusive relationship. This is particularly the case when one considers the parallels between the seductive and 'rewarding' nature of the abuse and very similar themes that are repeated in his heterosexual relationships.

There are a number of other references in the interview narratives that suggest that this object relationship forms part of a sophisticated defensive strategy. Importantly, the omnipotence gained from this sexualized experience also serves to defend against aggression or potential conflict. Here, gratification is obsessively sought in order to avoid the strong identification of being a weak 'spineless' man. Hate and aggression appears once this gratifying relationship is threatened in some way. Consistent with this, it appears that separation from this gratifying relationship turns the internal object into a threatening 'evil' object that evokes hatred and is attacked. In other words, it appears that the gratifying aspect of the original object relationship develops into a defensive strategy in an attempt to keep away bad parts of the original object.

The 'mysterious' attack has three important elements to it that strongly suggests that the above object constellation plays an important role in the murder. First, the separation, although not consciously acknowledged by him as important, is strongly linked to the source of his aggression in other instances. Second, the threatened withdrawal of 'gifts' appears to make him feel far more vulnerable than before. Finally, his inability to complete the sexual act because of his impotence seriously challenges his capacity to maintain or uphold his defensive system which, as we have seen, is based largely on a particular kind of gratification. All these threats were significantly over-determined by past relationships and appear linked to the collapse of a defensive system that Ben worked hard to uphold. With this, and bearing a striking resemblance to his dream, his internal representation of his girlfriend shifts to the hated, evil object that 'these females' always threaten to become.

With this general formulation in mind, I want now to consider the role of the final three dimensions of violence.

Brutalization of the self: trauma and loss

To what extent does trauma play a role in the actions of these offenders and how is it managed intrapsychically? Ben's prolonged exposure to sexual abuse clearly impacted on most of his behaviour throughout his life leading to him developing particular defensive strategies. We have already established that the true implications of trauma can only really be ascertained by understanding how its effects are internalized and what the nature of the 'total situation' is at the time. In other words, the traumatic incident cannot simply be viewed as a concrete object in itself with invariable traumatic implications for the show of aberrant behaviour or psychopathology. As mentioned earlier, clearly not all murderers are traumatized and not all victims of trauma inevitably turn to violence. What is more, whether trauma actually occurs, as in the case of Ben, in itself, does not help us understand the dynamics of the case further. How it becomes part of the internal world, its location and function, is a more incisive question.

In Ben's case, the abuse took place in a seductive, 'loving' and gratifying environment where he felt acknowledged and understood. The value of this to him appears to be what stops him from any display of anger towards his uncle. He essentially transfers this pattern on to his heterosexual relationships. Clearly here, sexual elements of his relationship are compulsive and over-determined in a way that creates a defensive form of gratification and self-acknowledgment. In short, sex, and the repetition of the initial trauma, had been appropriated as a means of keeping away an unbearable sense of shame and self-hate.

Whether childhood trauma of this kind is often evident in the case histories of rage-type murderers is a debatable issue. As the reader may have gathered from some of the other cases explored, sometimes there is little evidence of childhood trauma at all. Certainly, in my experience, severe childhood trauma as a result of sexual abuse or violence is not typical of this profile. I would say that offenders who have sustained significant brutalization more typically present with aggressive and psychopathic characteristics. This is consistent with a need to identify with the perpetrator in order to 'escape' feeling victimized by such horrors. In the cases I have considered, 'milder' signs of trauma have sometimes been evident, as in the case of Andrew and Simon, where its implications could be resisted without having to identify with the aggressor.

When past trauma is apparent in rage offenders it appears to take a particular form whereby aspects of the self exposed become strongly associated with the split-off bad-object system referred to earlier. The area of trauma remains relatively inaccessible and cannot easily be articulated, reflecting the extent to which traumatic experience is felt to be indigestible. As Hyatt-Williams (1998) points out, traumatic experience often exists in the psyche in an unmetabolized form as it is too difficult to tolerate the psychic pain involved in its assimilation. In Ben's case, it is clearly evident that trauma, above all other factors, is responsible for the formation of the defensive organization. The sexual abuse he sustained leads to the construction of a narcissistic exoskeleton that is based almost entirely on gratification of the object or self. It is idealized and sexualized within the context of this narcissistic structure, whilst the real damage is split off. The real impact, as hypothesized earlier, is felt only when Ben can no longer sustain the split, turning his good object into an 'evil' bad object, revealing the true impact of the trauma.

Although 'identification with the aggressor' is perhaps one of the key defensive means of dealing with indigestible traumatic experience, this does not appear to be the case with this group of offenders. There are few indications that a stable identification with a traumatizing object is formed. Perhaps this is understandable given the nature of the defensive system and the internal control it exercises over aggressive objects. Certainly, the rage attack itself might be understood as a sudden identification with the aggressor in cases where trauma clearly took place. But even in these cases, the attack does not appear to be perpetrated via an established or cohesive identification with the aggressor. Ben does not identify with his uncle as perpetrator. If he did one would expect to find signs of him assuming a more dominant role in the traumatic repetitions that played themselves out in relationships linked to his sexual encounters. But as we have seen, this is not the dominant defensive pattern. More generally, if this were the case, there would also be more evidence of a threatening, aggressive approach to matters, especially in cases where some form of aggression or violence was experienced. As we have seen, however, a more compliant and diminutive defensive style is most apparent in such cases.

The poor representational capacity evident in these cases also suggests that coherent identifications with hostile objects may be hampered. This is so if one agrees that adequate representational capacity is a necessary forerunner to the process of identification proper (Gaddini, 1992). As we shall see in more detail in the following chapter, the dynamic motivation for the attack is more about the elimination of traumatic or shameful experience and the restoration of an all-good object system.

Although I am in agreement with Hyatt-Williams about the indigestible nature of trauma when it occurs in these individuals, I do not see it as the key to understanding the psychodynamics of rage-type murder. He places great emphasis on traumatic consequences 'driving' the eventual eruption of violence. I differ in emphasis here in that I see the defensive organization, which may not always result from trauma, as primary. In terms of other dimensions too, we have seen that under-represented aspects of the psyche may result not only from trauma, but also from the need to perpetuate an idealized symbiotic relationship that creates chronic hypersensitivity to disapproval or other negative aspects of the object. It seems that the construction of the defensive organization may be supported by factors like over-stimulation and problems related to separation where parts of the self associated with parental need and symbiotic relating are idealized. This has the effect of fostering a phobic response towards anything that cannot be construed in this light. Anything contrary to this is perceived as threatening and toxic. Of course, by implication, and in line with Shengold's argument, this would mean that anything that is associated with the individual's own potential – the self not dependent on symbiotic relating – would be felt to be terrifyingly insufficient and shameful. Here, the core of what is resisted need not emanate from any obvious trauma, the entrenched defences are more directly linked to protection against the paralysing effects that the absence of self engenders in such individuals. It amounts to a situation where the core of the self is felt to be like a psychic 'black hole'. Here, absence is felt to be terrifying and all-consuming, with no defined beginning or end. Although Grant (p.131) was often the victim of his wife's anger, this appeared to be far outweighed by his dependence on an idealized image of their relationship through which little reason or reality could penetrate. This appeared to be a continuation of his relationship with his mother. From what I could establish there were no clear signs of trauma evident in his past that might account for the entrenched splitting apparent in his personality. What was evident, however, was a desperate sense of loneliness when faced with separations from either his wife or mother. He described it as a 'terrible feeling of emptiness and deadness' that made him feel suicidal at times. I think his experience here says something about how terrifying separation, and the sense of thinking about himself as separate, can be when idealization has promised so much. Extreme idealization, originating from symbiotic object relations, makes anything that is 'other' feel alien and terrifying.

In sum then, dimensions of violence like the defensive organization, representational capacity and the nature of object relating are not always dependent on traumatogenic factors – related to past trauma – in the cases I have explored.

As opposed to childhood trauma, contemporary events related to loss and trauma, although often denied by the offender, are always in some way evident in the build-up to the murder. Ben was unable to deal with the significance of the break up of his relationship which meant much more to him than he was able to recognize. Simon, on the other hand, was trying to shield himself from the real implications of his wife's affair. The effects of this kind of stress are difficult to understand as the consequences are not always apparent in the behaviour or recollections of the offender. In most cases of rage-type murder there is a sense that the cumulative effects of such incidents have a traumatic effect on the ego, threatening its ability to overcontrol in its usual fashion. But this process still remains largely unexpressed by the offender and is incubated in some way. In this way the offenders' aggression is often imperceptible to their victims.

It appears that contemporary trauma is an essential ingredient in the build-up to murderous action. Although it cannot account for why the offender would murder, such incidents render the individual vulnerable to such action. The pathway to murder is not an inevitability until such individuals find themselves embroiled in some form of crisis. Only here is their exposure to shame or 'badness' felt to be so devastating and destructive.

The trauma of the murder itself is worth considering briefly here because it appears to be dealt with in a way that is consistent with existing defensive strategies. In most cases the offender's murderousness is still experienced in a dissociated manner. It is still not felt to be a part of the self and thus cannot be mourned. We see this with Ben where he is unable really to feel the destructive consequences of his actions and he still finds himself wondering if he actually committed the act. In many ways, in fact, he leaves me with a sense that he still feels that she is alive.

The ability truly to mourn the destruction of the object requires a re-negotiation of the central split in the personality. In Andrew's case, in Chapter 6, we begin to see some progress in this regard. Here, some depressive experience is evident in his working through of his relationship with his father and consequent losses, as well as the implications of the murder itself. As a result, he seems better able to tolerate psychic pain and consequent mourning of the lost object. In most cases, however, depressive experience cannot be tolerated, a finding consistent with Hyatt-Williams' (1998) and Gallwey's (1985) work. The effect is that no *real* loss is experienced. Psychic change in the depressive position always involves some form of loss and mourning at an intrapsychic level to facilitate the transformation process. The fact that there is often little evidence of this appears to reflect the rigid and immobile nature of the object constellation that dominates psychological processes. As outlined earlier, the narcissistic manner in which offenders relate may also give the impression that trauma, bad experience, and the like, are being processed and mourned. There are few indications, however, that this is really engaged with. I referred to this earlier as a kind of pseudo or 'as if' digestive capacity.

The role of phantasy/fantasy

How we understand the phantasy/fantasy world of the offender has important implications for what we think goes on in the offender's mind prior to the murder. In what way does the propensity to murder exist in his or her conscious or unconscious mind prior to the incident?

I pointed out earlier that self-preservative violence has often been associated with phantasies related to an engulfing maternal object. Here, phantasies involving the maternal object revolve around a dilemma between fusion and separateness. Either way, the self is felt to be under threat of annihilation. This kind of dilemma was apparent in Ben's thinking about his victim who had come to represent both elements of the original traumatogenic object: maternal and caring on the one hand, yet evil and all-consuming on the other. He described his experience with her as follows:

> She made me feel like someone else, I could do things for her that made her happy ... But sometimes it felt like she was taking over me in a weird way, like I could not let go. I think we needed each other so much it was dangerous, when we were together we could not be apart or leave each other alone. And I suppose when we were apart it hurt like hell, like someone had taken from me, although I did not want her to know that so I played it cool.

His statement here seems to capture the all-consuming nature of their relationship as well as the pending destructiveness that always threatened. It suggests that either way, in phantasy, traces of annihilatory threats towards the self are present, in fusion and separation. This dilemma appears most evident with specific reference to the build-up to violence, to which we will return shortly. In addition, however, phantasies consistent with the structure of their defensive organization also appear to be of great significance here. Such phantasies strive rigidly to counter threats of annihilation or any exposure of what I have called the bad-object system.

One of the most prominent phantasies relates to the constant replenishment of good in the external/maternal object ultimately to ensure the survival of the self and to prevent the object from 'seeing' any bad in the self. Simon, for example, does this by constantly evoking an intact, idealized perception of his mother and desperately tries to relive this through his wife, no matter what the cost.

Often such phantasies are accompanied by a strong misguided and arrogant belief that the bad internal world has no impact on the offender's interaction with external objects. To return to the case of Ben; he essentially 'blinds' his object with obsessive sexual needs and the desire to 'serve'. He believes that he is protected from his own hostility and can do no wrong in his relationships with others as long as he maintains this role. A corollary of this relates to the unconscious belief that if 'badness' is taken into the self, or internalized, it will disappear and can be forgotten. Conflict or bad experience is not internalized for the purposes of assimilation and integration. It is more readily associated with a phantasy of removing bad experience from the external world in the hope that it would disappear. Reflecting on his history of abuse, Ben reasoned that he believed it was counterproductive to talk about what had happened to him. He felt that because he had never told anyone – apart from myself and a psychiatrist – he had almost forgotten it entirely. Grant, in the previous chapter, also demonstrated this kind of logic in talking about his religious faith. For him, religious practice helped him 'forget and only think of good things'. Later he told me, again in a rather unconvincing way, that religion 'was able to extinguish what was wrong'. I do not mean to imply here that religion, after a catastrophe of this nature, is always a defensive attempt to 'cover up' perceived bad in the self and disown responsibility for the crime. Indeed, in a number of cases I have worked with, religious faith can be an enormous resource in helping offenders move towards depressive experience where they are able to eventually mourn for lost or damaged objects – external objects and internal objects that make up parts of the self.

A related phantasy that often emerges through their actions is the idea that 'as long as you are good, you will never be exposed to bad'. Phantasies such as this are often used to justify actions. Such a belief would, of course, also render them much more vulnerable to feeling slighted or humiliated when something inevitably goes wrong.

The above phantasies, understood in terms of primary object relations, suggests a more mature structure than phantasies simply related to annihilation and an engulfing object, typical of the dilemmas related to fusion and separateness. In my view, the infant is less passive and maintains some control over the symbiotic relationship with the maternal object. Aggression and bad part-objects or sensations are split off and locked inside the infant away from the maternal object. In a particular way, Biven's (1977) observations related to the individual 'borrowing as it were, the strength and cohesiveness from a more powerful object ' (p.351), resonates with these findings. The cohesiveness of the external object, in phantasy, is relied on here to confirm further the existence of a good external world, in turn confirming that it is different and separate from the internal bad world.

Importantly, there is little evidence that these individuals are plagued by phantasies of violence and destructiveness. This is often observed to be a typical pattern in most violent individuals (Biven, 1997; Meloy, 1992; Satten *et al.*, 1960). Earlier I referred to such a case, the case of Mark (p.44), where destructive phantasies clearly dominate the psyche. This man had endured a considerable bout of brutalization as a child and his phantasy world vividly bore the scars. Such phantasies also held within them a recipe for violence where a single direct line between phantasy and violent action could be witnessed. His dreams were littered with scenes of destruction and war where he was the only lasting survivor. He was always clothed in full combat gear looking for those who had caused damage, but there were never any other human figures present, dead or alive. These images seemed clearly to reflect the state of Mark's internal world where threat and destruction had annihilated all human contact, and now he would strive to do the same. In offenders like Mark, such phantasies dominate all experience and can easily be observed in their general aggressive approach towards others.

Although the above is an extreme case, this kind of destructiveness is not discernible in rage offenders. If this were the case, one would expect to encounter many more references to destructive interchanges between the self and internal/external objects. There are, however, signs of destructiveness in some cases, suggesting a particular kind of phantasy structure. Here, a superior grandiose object, with which the offender identifies, launches internal attacks on objects associated with emotional pain and a consequent unbearable sense of shame. The phantasy thus appears to be related to the destruction of a vulnerable 'feeling' part of the self that is closely associated with the bad-object system. Ben, for example, could not allow himself to explore his own sense of shame and embarrassment. Rather, he took to telling me about how emotions and emotional people essentially feel like obstacles to him that he needed to 'shut down' or control in some way. He also described times when he would meet up with women and experience great embarrassment for no obvious reason. When this happened he would break off contact and castigate himself over the vulnerability he felt.

Turning to conscious fantasy, it appears that very few offenders experience aggressive or murderous fantasies directly related to the murder prior to the act. Although in some cases fantasies of wanting to act aggressively were evident, offenders who fit the 'overcontrolled' personality profile discussed earlier do not appear to experience clearly defined fantasies of murder prior to the act. My observations here differ from those put forward by Hyatt-Williams who believes that fantasies of murder are repeated several times in the offender's mind before they are eventually enacted on the physical world.

A far more prominent fantasy prior to the murder relates to a fear of being attacked. Here, the unmasking of the bad-object world, seen mirrored in external objects, is experienced as sudden, uncontrollable, and therefore extremely threatening. But why should it be that these offenders do not generally experience conscious fantasies of murder? Indeed, as we have already observed, these kinds of offenders often express a wish that they had entertained such fantasies. They believe that if this were the case, they would have been able to prevent the attack as such thoughts would have served as a warning sign of some kind. The absence of conscious fantasies of aggression appears to be best explained by the nature of the defensive system where potential aggressiveness is kept away from external reality and consciousness.

In sum then, unlike Satten *et al.*'s (1960) findings that these rage offenders usually have a primitive and violent fantasy life, I have not found this to be the case. My observations indicate that no clearly formulated and focused phantasies/fantasies of attack are present in such individuals. In other words, the intention to kill, as present in fantasy content, is not a key factor in influencing the course of events in these murders. This differs greatly from most murderer profiles where fantasy is usually present and is often one of the key determinants of a violent outcome.

It is worth noting that the above observations have important implications for considering the issue of criminal responsibility in rage-type murder. How should we determine the offender's criminal responsibility if they do not have conscious fantasies or intentions of killing? Minutiae of experience such as this are not often considered in evaluating cases of this kind. Understandably, they are dismissed as subjective hearsay and the reality of such claims is difficult to establish. Nevertheless, the absence of murderous fantasies has been a consistent finding in my work and cannot be dismissed as it informs our understanding of the motives and behaviour of these kinds of offender. I do not wish to enter into a debate here about how this might relate to the notion of criminal responsibility. I refer the reader to Goreta (1990) who provides a useful review of factors to be considered in assessing criminal responsibility from a psychoanalytical perspective.

I posed a question earlier about whether one would be able to pinpoint differences between fantasies that may be acted out and those that are not. This still remains difficult to answer and much work is still required here. We know, however, that it is less about the fantasy *per se* and more about the psychic context in which it occurs. Ego-syntonic homicidal fantasies, for instance, are much closer to action than ego-dystonic ones. The differences between psychopathic fantasies and obsessional fantasies represent extreme positions here. But this is of little use to us given that homicidal fantasies are not often apparent or conscious in rage offenders. Here other dimensions of violence, particularly the individual's defensive pattern, representational capacity and external situation, appear greatly to influence the outcome. I shall only briefly explore some of the possibilities open to consideration here. In the case of Grant, a case where some aggressive fantasy was experienced, the offender had endured a long history of strife and abuse. This appears to have been a key factor that eventually forces him to enact an extreme version of his fantasy. In exploring the defensive system most readily associated with rage, we also know that fantasy is not used as a vehicle for 'expulsion' and action, as is usually the case in typical borderline personalities. As we have seen, the ability to *re*-present fantasy and articulate it in a way that gives the individual some psychological distance will also influence that pathway to action. Finally, the chronicity of fantasies of being attacked by others and their relationship to specific external factors may also influence enactment. It is likely, for instance, that fantasies of persecution, experienced over a long period of time, and then confirmed by some shameful external happening, would render the individual much more vulnerable to a defensive violent response. The above are just some of the factors worth considering. Questions related to the pathways to action, via fantasy, still require further research before we are able to understand this process in greater detail.

Sexuality

Acts of violence observed here are not motivated by any direct primitive sexual need such as is found in sado-masochistic violence or perverse violence. Although sexual themes dominate in Ben's case, they do not enter the crime scene in a way that sexualizes the offence. Sexual acts had come to represent a primitive source of gratification, partly emerging as the re-enactment of a seductive and abusive relationship. The sexualization of his object relations, however, does not directly motivate aggression. Rather, the object constellation acts as a vehicle through which narcissistic reflection can occur as a defensive strategy. In other words, sexual needs serve the same function as the excessive and extravagant gift giving that occurs between victim and offender.

Often, however, salient themes related to sexual activity, normal or deviant, do not appear to be prominent in such cases. If one accepts the structure of the defensive organization proposed here, it is most likely that sexual and sensual excitation are experienced as chaotic and disruptive. Pleasurable sexual or sensual excitation requires that the offender relinquish aspects of his overcontrolling defensive system. Given its importance, however, it is likely that the overcontrolled offender would have great difficulty doing so. This seems to be the case unless it is incorporated into the defensive system itself where it becomes a means of perpetuating a narcissistic ideal, as in Ben's case.

Perelberg's (1999b) observations regarding the precarious nature of masculine identifications in violent men appears to take hold in a specific way in rage-type murderers. Grant gives us a sense of his experience of men and its impact on his sense of self in the following brief extract:

> There have never really been men in my life. My father yes, he provided for us but I never knew what I needed to do to follow him ... in his footsteps. We never had problems, maybe that's a bad thing, I don't know. I would try and do things like him, like sport, but I never felt good. Although, my father wasn't around much anyway, I preferred to do things for my mother anyway. I was mum's boy, as they used to say. But I had to grow up strong so I could eventually leave her ... In a way, I do wish I could stand up to them [men] more. I feel less about myself that I have to feel that way.

As in a number of cases I have worked with, Grant gives a sense that his own masculinity has had to develop in relative isolation from a paternal figure, leaving him more dependent on maternal objects. A precarious sense of masculinity thus develops in relation to the maternal object and the absence of the father and is less about conflict and rivalry with his father. As a result, oedipal experience is somewhat stunted. Masculinity is associated more with attempting to be separate from the maternal object than it is a symbol of virility and rivalry.

For Ben, the situation is more complicated. In the absence of significant parental figures, his uncle appears to become a bizarre conglomeration of maternal and paternal experience where he is perceived as not only caring, and nurturing, but also sexually stimulating. At the same time, he represents Ben's closest paternal figure. As a result he is left confused by a feminized masculine figure that causes all sorts of conscious and unconscious fears related to homosexuality. He was emphatic about his hate for homosexuals. Although I have emphasized the defensive function of his sexual relationships with women, it appears that his motivations here are over-determined. His behaviour also appears to have been a reaction formation against homosexual abusive fears that, at the same time, attempt to assert a fickle masculinity. Ben's avoidance of relating to men and his perception of their motives also sheds some light on his sense of masculinity. As Ben put it:

> Men are a weak species, they take what they want from each other and don't stand tall ... I suppose that means me too. But I tried to live my own independent life and didn't listen to other men. Women seemed to like that about me ... I'm not sure if that makes me a real man or what?

I did not answer the above question. But afterwards he appeared remarkably embarrassed for reasons that he could not state. His statements about his own masculinity – perhaps in relation to his perceptions of me – appeared to have precipitated a degree of insecurity and shame.

The precarious nature of masculine identifications appears to contribute to the vulnerability and defensiveness of these offenders when under threat. This is precisely Bromberg's argument, where violence erupts as a defensive response to sexual inadequacy and conflict. But the full thrust of what occurs internally appears to be closer to his initial formulation where the main vulnerability emerges, at a more primitive level, out of a perceived annihilation of the self where oral aggression dominates. We shall see how this occurs when we reconstruct some of the psychic processes that appear to underlie the act itself in the next chapter.

To continue, however, this does not mean that rivalrous challenges or sexual jealousy, as typical oedipal triggers, would not impact on these individuals or even precipitate violence. As argued earlier, oedipal and preoedipal psychic processes do not operate to the exclusion of each other. They should rather be understood as different 'registers' of experience, where one dominates the other, depending on the individual and his situation. When one scrutinizes the phenomenology of the experience reported here, such encounters are experienced as annihilatory in the extreme and there is little room for typical oedipal themes to be entertained or thought about in usual conflictual ways. Put another way, and referring back to the dynamics of rage, the offender's internal world is typically self-centred. Given this, object-oriented thought, the capacity to acknowledge the complexity and independence of the object, and the conflict that this inevitably brings, is mostly evaded.

In further support of this, typical countertransference–transference paradigms that emerge in working with rage offenders may also be understood as emerging out of a self-centred narcissistic orientation, although they often appear to be oedipal in nature. Often, these men spend a great deal of time overstating their achievements and successes along with a curiosity about the therapist's own accomplishments. A similar theme may also emerge when the patient places himself in 'competition' with the stated goals and achievements of therapy. These occurrences may easily be interpreted along oedipal lines as sensitivities towards masculine rivalry. But in the context of their defensive organizations, such statements, at their core, are better understood as being attempts to establish a narcissistic transference with a maternal object. Here, the therapist is needed to idealize masculine accomplishments so as to shield any recognition of potential conflict or the uncovering of his own shame.

Chapter 9

The act revisited

We return now to the act itself, hopefully with a better understanding of the premorbid personality and the psychodynamic processes most apparent in rage offenders. In this short chapter I want to consolidate my understanding of the sequence of dynamic events which eventually amount to murder. Making inferences about the sequence of events, internal and external, is of course complicated by the fact that few offenders are able to give a clear and coherent account of the situation. Even if their recollection appears reasonably clear, the accuracy of the account still needs to be questioned. For this reason, although I have been most interested in the offenders' subjective accounts of the murder, I have used police reports, the court's reconstruction of the crime and, where possible, witness accounts, to corroborate their recollections.

I have chosen the case of Philip to illustrate my findings here because he was able to provide me with the most vivid description of events. He described his emotional state that day in the following way: ' It was like an explosion waiting to happen. Like bad energy building up inside me that I didn't really know about. I knew there was something wrong but I didn't know what.' As alluded to earlier, the way Philip describes the surge of rage that accompanied the murder can readily be understood as being precipitated by a violent cathartic release. The idea of catharsis leaves one with an image of a repressed murderous part of the personality waiting to erupt once the ego is forced into a fragile position. As seen earlier, however, focusing solely on the build-up of affect runs the risk of obscuring the complexity of the interactional process that occurs during the murder. It also creates a false distinction between affective processes and underlying object relations. Following Kernberg (1984), I have previously argued that affect is always a product of the emotional valences carried between particular object relations. With this in mind, let us consider Philip's case in more detail. I shall confine myself to limited detail about his history and focus more on the act itself.

PHILIP

Philip was a 29-year-old Indian man. He was the youngest in his family and had 2 brothers 8 and 10 years older. When he was a young child, his father worked as a tax consultant whilst his mother remained at home. He described himself as being very close to his mother, and as the youngest child, he would get most of the attention. Philip always saw his father as being close to his older brothers and felt that he had little time for him. Their relationship appeared to be characterized by indifference. Although he could not articulate it, it appears that Philip felt considerable resentment towards his father for 'neglecting' him. His father died from a heart attack when Philip was 17 years old. Although he was worried about how his mother would cope with his father's death, Philip felt relatively unmoved by the event.

Shortly after his father's death, Philip left home to study engineering at university. It was clear to him at this point that he would need to work hard at his studies so he would be able to return home and support his mother. Whilst at university he managed to obtained a bursary and used much of this money to support his mother and eldest brother.

After his studies he returned home and found employment nearby. He remained with this company for 5 years and had become very popular and successful during this period. He was known to work long hours and would make sure his senior colleagues acknowledged his contribution. Philip was described as a diligent worker who was often commended by his seniors for his high standard of work.

He kept a number of friends, although he felt it better to describe them as 'acquaintances' as he felt he was never able to talk to them about himself. He had had a number of short sexual relationships with women which were discontinued for similar reasons. It was clear to him that he preferred to be at home with his mother and had little interest in pursuing other relationships.

Philip's situation changed considerably after a particular incident at work. He had happened to make a mistake in his calculations for a job quotation. This led to him being called in by a senior colleague who reprimanded him for overspending. He found this very difficult to accept and felt defeated by his actions. He found it difficult to continue working and withdrew from many of his activities at work. Feeling unappreciated, he began entertaining thoughts of leaving his job and seeking employment elsewhere. His demeanour was clearly apparent to others. One particular colleague described him as having 'a personality change' after the problem had arisen. Despite these obvious changes, Philip took to convincing himself that 'nothing had really happened' and that things had returned to normal.

Approximately 3 weeks later, in an unrelated incident, Philip had an altercation with a neighbour who had parked in his parking bay. He described this neighbour as a 'friend' who 'admired [him] for achieving so much'. In this instance, however, the man contested his claim about the parking and insulted him for being so persistent. Enraged by this, Philip struck the man several times. At this point it appears that his victim attempted to flee but was again overpowered by Philip. This time he repeatedly beat his head against a kerb until he lay motionless. Realizing what he had done, he attempted to hide the body and fled the scene. Two hours later he returned and handed himself over to the police and accompanied the police to the crime scene. Medical reports showed that his victim died from multiple head injuries caused by repeated blows delivered with considerable force.

Throughout my interviews with Philip he adopted a forced obligatory manner that engendered in me a sense that he was doing me a great favour in being interviewed. One of the most apparent features of his interviews was his non-verbal approach. He often appeared startled and shameful or embarrassed about what he was saying, checking with me to see if it were correct. However, he denied any embarrassment and, instead, would often reply by 'agreeing' that he too had noticed how easily others were embarrassed. He appeared to equate emotional vulnerability with weakness and often chastised others for dwelling on their emotions.

Two core identifications emerged in my interviews with Philip, one superior and somewhat grandiose, the other threatened, ashamed and largely unconscious. As is typical of the 'narcissistic exoskeleton', the 'superior' identification relates to the part of himself associated with shame, violence and suffering in a harsh and demeaning way. This dominant sense of identity worked to split off emotional experience by attacking it in this way.

A substantial portion of Philip's object world appeared to be based on the avoidance of shame. Indeed objects associated with shame and suffering lacked any clear representational definition. As with some of the other cases I have explored, this appeared to be part of a defensive attempt to preserve an unfaltering self-image.

I turn now to considering the sequence of dynamic events that appears best to explain the act itself. I shall use Philip's rather candid recollections to illustrate my understanding.

Weakening of the narcissistic exoskeleton

When I think about it now I can't understand how work had got so bad. Yes there was that problem at work but I didn't hate anyone, I just felt unappreciated. Still it affected the way I saw my life, somehow it lost meaning, it knocked me. Sometimes I think I was depressed but I didn't tell and tried not to show anyone, I didn't really feel it myself and pretended it wasn't happening.

The murderous event usually begins long before the actual attack with the persistent challenging of the defensive organization. This need not necessarily occur within the victim–offender relationship, as is the case with Philip.

In most cases I have explored, conflict most commonly emerges in response to themes of separation or antagonism linked to the external object. From this point on the victim becomes a threat to the offender's defensive armour. Because of the nature of the defensive system itself, however, much of the impact of the conflict is denied. Only in his reconstruction of events is Philip able to recognize his depressive reaction and the unconscious hostility present in him at the time. Attempts at denial essentially begin to fail along with the weakening exoskeleton. Because the offender's identity is almost solely based on the defensive system, he begins to feel increasingly threatened by his own inner turmoil.

With the defensive system weakened, the offender is forced to face an internal crisis where the existence of neglected unarticulated parts of the self can no longer be split off with effective rigidity. From our previous analysis we know that this part of the self largely lacks any representational capacity in the psyche. In Bion's (1962b) terms, it exists as a system of β-elements unelaborated by thought, leaving the offender with no means of articulating his distress. Along with the weakening of defences the boundaries between self and other, internal and external, begin to diminish leading to a growing sense of confusion. This is more typical of chronic catathymia where there exists a period of incubation in which the individual struggles with his own inner turmoil before it leads to murder.

The final provocation and the collapse of the defensive system

> When he said 'fuck you', I lost it and felt there was no way out. It was like I had lost myself actually and become numb to everything around me ... Something snapped and told me that it would never be the same again ... He was my neighbour, a friend. We had never fought before, but at that moment it was like he was someone else, a kind of danger to my life who would not hear what I was saying.
>
> I can see it now, it was like it would never end. I just got sucked into it without thinking.

Given the poor representational capacity of the psyche the final provocation is experienced as a devastating attack on the self. It cannot be subject to thought and consequently overwhelms the offender and his defensive system. The collapse of the defences magnifies the intrusive experience to a point where it becomes life threatening.

Some of the trigger events are 'objectively' intimidating. Philip was involved in an explosive altercation. In Andrew's case, someone known to be aggressive threatened him. But why are these experienced as life threatening? There appear to be two reasons. First, at an intrapsychic level the victim-to-be is a key object in the offender's defensive system. The defensive system cannot function without the victim's compliance in confirming or mirroring the existence of the 'ideal' self.

The provocation by the victim-to-be thus triggers in the offender a sudden loss of self-identity. Of course, this may occur by displacement where the victim is equated with those threatening his defensive hold on reality. Unbeknown to Philip's neighbour, his challenging of Philip's position is equated with the seething turmoil he had been experiencing for a number of weeks. In doing so the victim-to-be also breaks with his perceived role as 'admirer', essentially confirming the collapse of the narcissistic exoskeleton.

Second, with the collapse of the defensive system, all that had been defensively internalized, split off and 'forgotten', is suddenly thrust to the foreground of the personality. It is probable that, at this moment, the ideal self is felt to have been annihilated and replaced by bad internalized objects. In sum, the sudden loss of this part of the self and its replacement with unmanageable experience appears to explain why these threats are felt to be so deadly. This process can clearly be observed as re-enacted in Ben's dream, discussed in the previous chapter. In his dream he is engaged in sexual contact with his 'ideal' lover, but once she stops telling him how good he is – the lapse in the defensive system – she turns into an 'evil-devil-thing' – a symbol of the dangerous bad-object system.

As suggested earlier, the collapse of the defensive system may also expose the offender to a terrifying sense of absence, a 'black hole', akin to the sudden loss or death of the self. In these instances, as I think was the case with Philip, it is not so much the presence of traumatizing bad internal objects that prompts distress, it is more that the bad-object system is, at its core, based on an annihilatory sense of absence that threatens to be all-consuming.

The thrust at which the bad-object system is felt to contaminate the self is of great importance here. The speed at which the murderous interchange occurs certainly lessens the chances of any psychic digestion occurring. More importantly, however, and as alluded to earlier, the bad-object system comprises mainly destructive paranoid experience and is synonymous with the suspension of the Ps $\leftrightarrow D$ process of psychic digestion (Bion, 1962b). Once the defensive system collapses, a surge of persecutory anxiety is felt to overwhelm the psyche making psychic digestion a near impossibility as most objects are perceived as extremely threatening. It is probable that any attempts at containment, at this stage, would be experienced as dangerously entrapping rather than comforting. The incubation period of this highly dissociated state varies depending on the specifics of the situation. Furthermore, the extent to which the murderous exchange is, in part, precipitated by the victim's violent projective identifications, as discussed in Chapter 7, also depends on the nature of the case.

Intrusive identification with the bad object

It was almost like I needed to become someone else, someone who could be violent because he was acting aggressively. He started it, I still think that. He was pushing me into it. I had never been aggressive but it was like I was schizophrenic, I just snapped into a mad state and I couldn't stop.

As the above statement suggests, the collapse of the narcissistic exoskeleton is followed by identification with the bad object which is experienced as being forced into the offender by the victim. This, in turn, activates a parallel internal crisis involving the previously encapsulated part of the self. With the 'ideal' self destroyed and with no experience of good supportive objects accessible to him at that moment, he has no option but to identify with the bad-object system. This is apparent in some of the other cases we have considered. Andrew, in a split second, is forced to identify with his ex-partner's aggressive statement that, in turn, resonates with his own split-off bad objects. Ralph, on the other hand, clearly remembered thinking that he was about to die. Here again, there is a forced identification with a persecuted object. Swamped by persecutory experience it is also likely at this point that the offender is overwhelmed by indigestible fantasies of death in the way that Hyatt-Williams (1998) has suggested.

There is another element to this momentary lapse that appears to add to the escalation of the explosive situation. There are indications that the identification, in turn, evokes an unbearable sense of shame and humiliation in the offender. As discussed earlier, shame is directly associated with the internalized bad-object system. I use the term here to characterize a state of 'defenseless exposure' evident just after the moment of provocation when the defensive system is breached. Shame, in part, appears associated with exposure to indigestible aspects of the self that have resulted from trauma. As we have seen, Grant, Ben and Andrew all associate feelings of shame with trauma. They re-experience this in an intoxicating form just prior to the crime. As Hyatt-Williams puts it, the reaction is analogous to an allergic response where a particular sensitivity is activated. In some of the cases explored, there are clear indications that the offender's violence is a defensive reaction towards the repetition of a traumatic object constellation. We could understand Andrew's reaction, for instance, as being a response to re-encountering his father in his victim. Ben's actions also appear strongly linked to a distorted repetition of the abuse he had endured. In my view, however, it is not always the case that the repetition of an encapsulated trauma triggers murderous action.

Even when there is little sign of trauma, such as in Philip's case, these individuals often present as being very vulnerable to shameful exposure. It appears that the forced identification with the bad-object system magnifies this residual sense of shame to an unbearable extreme, forcing the individual into violence. Shengold's (1991) description of the rage reaction as being evoked by a shameful loss of what the self represents appears fitting here. In his terms, it is felt to be a sudden collapse of 'everything' and the daunting exposure of the self as 'nothing', the ultimate narcissistic injury. He links this to the sudden loss of narcissistic forms of relating: what I have called the narcissistic exoskeleton here and what Ruoloto (1968) terms the 'pride system'. The nature of the explosive rage that occurs in response to the collapse of more adaptive defences appears consistent with those who have argued that rage is essentially a primitive defensive response to 'excessive unpleasure' (Parens, 1993). Often, the sense of shame that initiates the rage attack is also linked to fears of annihilation or death of the self.

Evacuation via projective identification and annihilation of the bad object in the victim

> I attacked him because he was forcing me to, he was not leaving me alone and he was making me aggressive. This sounds crazy, and what I did was wrong, but in that moment it was like I had to end it otherwise it would go on forever and I would not been seen as the right one in the argument. We would have both been wrong.

The intolerable, life-threatening nature of this internal state leaves the offender little option but to project it outwards. Philip's statement aptly describes this process whereby he is desperate to unburden himself in order to 'escape' the situation and his own internal chaos. Ironically, the fantasy of projection and annihilation of the object is an attempt to see himself as 'right' in the argument and exonerated from any sense of shame. In the final devastating move in this sequence, the bad object is destroyed in the victim in a frenzy proportionate to the devastation that the offender has felt internally. As in most cases, the projective identification used here is not dispersive; it is aimed specifically at where the distress was perceived to have come from. In this sense, these acts of rage-type murder differ from psychotic acts of violence (Blackburn, 1993; Sohn, 1995).

The eruption is more than simply a cathartic release. It is perpetuated by a desperate need to annihilate the bad object and the psychic pain it causes. This is in keeping with Meloy's (1992) and Hyatt-Williams' (1998) observations. It is important to note that in many cases the sequence of events described thus far does not occur in a simple linear fashion. As I alluded to earlier, often the victim and offender engage in a terrifying juggling of indigestible psychic states where the boundaries between victim and offender no longer clearly show themselves. Whether this occurs or not would depend largely on the nature of *situational factors* and how they impact on the intrapsychic dimensions of violence.

Re-establishment of the defensive system

> Afterwards I was shocked. I told myself I must think like a criminal and hide the body but I eventually came to my mind and gave myself up. I struggle to feel anything about what I did. Others are embarrassed about what I did. I don't think about it and try and live life the best I can. When I wake it is hard to feel that I did it.

After the murder, the offender is typically traumatized by his own actions as well as by the overwhelming nature of previously dissociated experience. In some cases an impulsive reaction follows where there is an attempt to cover up the killing or to flee the scene. It may be that, whilst the offender is still in a dissociated state, these actions resemble a last-ditch attempt at reinstating the defensive system and defensively 'covering up' the damaged object. Andrew's case (Chapter 6) illustrates this well, where he buries the body in a field associated with his childhood, a representation of his previously abandoned bad objects. Of course, this process has little effect on the reality of the situation. When the offender emerges from his dissociated state he is left to face the daunting realization that his distressed psychic state has been irreversibly imprinted on his real external objects.

The way Philip describes his actions, however, suggests that there may also be a different motivation behind such behaviour. His statement suggests that the 'cover-up' emanates from a continued identification with the bad-object system where he needs to 'think like a criminal'. Here, he appears to make an attempt to identify with a psychic state not usually available to him. It is only afterwards, when he hands himself over, that this shifts. It is often difficult to say which of these above motivations dominate. What is clear, however, is that shortly after the murder some sense of reality is quickly restored. The defensive organization, the exoskeleton, however, takes some time to be restored as the individual is hampered by constant reminders of his 'evil' actions.

In my experience it is not always the case that the offender experiences a sense of relief in the aftermath of the attack. Usually the offender continues to be haunted and traumatized by his or her actions for sometime afterwards. In the aftermath of the murder he or she is forced to confront a disowned part of him- or herself and constantly oscillates between belief and disbelief in this part. That is, until his or her narcissistic defences are eventually restored. If a sense of relief is experienced, it appears to be linked to the unconscious belief that the offender's actions have succeeded in evacuating and destroying the bad-object system. Affective discharge accompanies this process, but is not divorced from accompanying object relations.

After the murder it often appears that the defensive organization returns with even greater rigidity whereby compliance, over-obligation and phantasies of reinstating 'good' in their objects are held up with a conviction to 'seek forgiveness'. Although I do not doubt that sometimes some degree of reparation is present in these actions, it most often resembles a kind of manic reparation where previously disowned parts of the self are split off with even greater force.

Chapter 10

Some thoughts on assessment, treatment and prevention

We are faced with a number of problems in assessing and treating rage-type offenders. Many of these problems are related to the encapsulated nature of the rage offender's personality. The characteristics of the personality, the act and related intrapsychic dimensions have a number of implications for assessment, treatment and prevention. Before outlining some of the prominent issues here, I shall recapitulate key points raised in the investigation.

I have been interested in rage-type offenders who usually have no significant history of violence, are described as being ostensibly 'normal' and are often successful in their achievements. I have argued that this is best understood as being part of a rigid defensive pattern and is not simply about the relative 'normality' of everything when compared to murder or extreme rage. Given the overcontrolling nature of the personality, symptoms of distress are usually masked and overt signs of psychopathology are often absent. The lack of motive and the sudden explosive nature of the offence make the act especially difficult to understand.

Two observations have been consistently reported in this area of research: first, offenders are often reported to have a borderline personality organization. Second, the act is ultimately described as being defensive in nature. The broad use of the term 'borderline personality' in the literature often makes it difficult to understand how the borderline pattern is implicated in different forms of violence. Frequently the borderline personality is referred to, either by name or description, with little reference to the numerous different dynamic constellations that may occur in the offender. I have argued that a particular type of overcontrolling borderline personality appears to describe best the structural aspects of the rage offender's internal world. My observations suggest that careful distinction between different borderline patterns and their corresponding violent presentations are required in order to understand intrapsychic motivations for violence.

In exploring the dimensions of rage-type murder, the defensive organization appears best to elucidate the core dynamics behind the aberrant reaction and its defensive nature. Although it is well established that the act itself is essentially defensive on a psychological level, my analysis has attempted to show the extent to which the defensiveness of the final aberrant act has long been deeply entrenched in the personality, forming a narcissistic exoskeletal-type structure.

This defensive edifice comprises good idealized objects and encapsulated bad objects that are held apart by rigid splitting defences. The exoskeleton has two essential features. First, splitting occurs in a particular way whereby the fantasy of the external world as being an all-good reflection of the self is rigidly maintained, forming a defensive shield around the personality. As we have seen, this does not mean that such individuals are not exposed to bad experience in reality or that they are not unconsciously 'motivated' to invite bad experience or conflict into their lives. It is the *fantasy* of 'goodness' that needs to be upheld at all costs. Earlier, I discussed a number of ways in which the defensive system manipulates the object world to ensure that the all-good self is maintained despite being confronted with real conflict. The kind of defensive strategies employed here share a number of similarities with the way false self pathology and the 'as if' personality have been conceptualized.

The second feature of the defensive organization relates to the defensive internalization of bad objects further to preserve the all-good 'external' world. As a consequence, the 'internal' world, in phantasy, is largely disowned as it becomes the vessel for compacted, internalized bad-object relations – the bad-object system – associated with aggression. It is ironic, of course, that what is 'designed' to defend the personality against bad experience, through internalization, is also precisely what leaves these offenders vulnerable to committing rage-type murder.

In the cases explored here there is little evidence that rage-type murder is propelled solely by a death impulse that eventually erupts when ego functioning is vulnerable. This is not to say, however, referring back to my central argument in Chapter 4, that other forms of violence do not more readily fit this pattern. The rage constellation, as conceptualized here, is primarily a last-ditch attempt to preserve the self and is not motivated by a preconceived 'wish' to destroy the object. The attack is better explained as having its origins in the defensive processes of the psyche. As Glasser (1998) points out, the fate of the object is less significant in preservative forms of violence. Emphasis is on survival of the self. Destruction of the object, as tragic as it is in the reality of the situation, is only a secondary consequence.

I have also shown how other prominent dimensions appear to take on a particular form that is consistent with the defensive system. The bad-object system, for instance, appears to be more closely associated with the part of the personality that has a poor representational capacity. Paternal and maternal representations have been understood as being allied with specific areas of the defensive system, contributing to its structure. Still further, the way trauma is internalized and associated with the bad object also appears to add to this kind of defensive structure.

It is important to reiterate that I am not suggesting here that all assaults or murders committed during a bout of rage have the same psychodynamic pattern. Earlier, in Aggression, Rage and Violence (Chapter 1), I argued for a clear distinction between different acts of violence and corresponding personality characteristics in order to avoid such an oversimplification. Clearly, more overtly destructive personality types, not fitting the definition of the rage-type murderer outlined here, are equally capable of committing rage offences (Revitch and

Schlesinger, 1981; Roth, 1990). The psychodynamics and meaning behind such rage acts committed in different contexts – internal and external – would be very different from that of rage-type murder. Some of these differences evident in the literature have been pointed out in Seven Intrapsychic Dimensions of Violence (Chapter 2).

Although emphasis has been on how intrapsychic factors contribute towards the propensity to commit a murderous act, these cannot be considered in isolation of effects external to the individual. Such influences would include immediate stressors, the actions of the victim, and the nature of events that surround the build-up to the offence. Similarly, there is little doubt that broader external factors – social, cultural and environmental – also have a role to play in this kind of offence. For instance, one might argue that a number of the murders discussed earlier may not have taken place if firearms were not so easily available or sought after. Perhaps, we could argue, the offenders' rage would have had less tragic consequences if a firearm were not available. A lot more could be said about the interaction between internal and external factors here and indeed it remains an important area of research.

Assessment of dangerousness

The careful assessment of a potential offender, should they be seen by a health care professional, is, of course, the first step to preventing violence. More often, however, assessment occurs following the crime, as a means of establishing a psychological profile for forensic and legal purposes.

In the case of the former type of assessment, much has been written about the problems involved in assessing dangerousness and opinions differ on the validity of actuarial and clinically based models of prediction (Blackburn, 1993; Bottoms, 1982; Cox, 1982; Farrington and Gunn, 1985; Glasser, 1996; Hinton, 1983). Most, however, agree that the best 'predictor' of potential violence is a previous history of violence. This, of course, is of little help when it comes to the rage-type offender who, by definition, has no significant history of violence. The apparent 'normality' of these individuals and their 'as if' way of dealing with conflict further complicates the assessment of potential violence.

In terms of the actual build-up to the incident, however, it is worth distinguishing between acute and chronic catathymia. In chronic catathymia the murderous intention is more easily detected in the incubation phase where signs of dissociation and distress are more overt. It appears, for instance in Ralph's case, that catathymic turmoil was overtly apparent to others around him despite nothing being done about it. When the action is acute, however, there is much less chance of identifying potential offenders. This is where observations regarding the intrapsychic world of the offender may be particularly useful. Factors making the individual more vulnerable to rage are summarized as follows.

a)   A situation where signs of escalating conflict, often related to the loss of an object, are apparent but are minimized or denied by the offender.

b) The presence of a defensive organization that is characterized by the disavowal of bad, conflictual experience and the presence of an idealized good-object system that is identified with as a means of reaffirming an all-good self. Over-obliging and submissive strategies, in order to avoid implicating the self in the conflict, may often be a part of the organization.

c) Evidence of an entrapping dyadic situation often experienced by rage offenders where little internal space is allocated to a 'third object'.

d) The presence of an attacking internal object associated with fantasies of being attacked or thoughts of suicide. Although not always the case, the attacking object may be reflected and reaffirmed in the external situation in which the individual finds himself.

e) The presence of precarious male identifications.

f) Indications of a poor representational capacity.

g) Evidence of trauma, past or present, that has not undergone a process of psychic digestion and instead becomes associated with the bad-object system.

h) Hypersensitivity to a sense of shame. Evidence of shameful experience harboured by the individual that is related to a fear of the bad-object system being exposed.

In addition to the above areas, it is also important for the clinician to assess whether there have been any sudden changes in the offender's libidinal organizations, whether the offender has alternative sources of self-esteem available to him, and the degree of flexibility he displays in altering interpersonal functioning (Cox, 1982).

It should be pointed out that one needs to be cautious in inferring any direct causal links between the above intrapsychic factors and the act itself. Assessment models of dangerousness often fall prey to simplistic assumptions regarding causal links between personality features and violence (Blackburn, 1993; Bottoms, 1982; Cox, 1982; Farrington and Gunn, 1985; Glasser, 1996; Hinton, 1983). This usually leads to gross over-predictions of dangerousness with little consideration being given to the dynamic complexities of the case. The idea of a 'profile' of the violent offender has unfortunately become associated with this kind of one-to-one deterministic reasoning. It is for this reason that I have deliberately avoided referring to the intrapsychic factors explored here as a 'profile' of the rage-type murderer. These dimensions, I would argue, should be viewed more as vulnerability factors that need to be considered in relation to one another in the context of the particular situation at hand. It is how these factors come together, specific to each case, which determines the offender's propensity to act violently.

In some cases, for instance, the indigestible nature of traumatic experience combined with the rigid defensive structure observed here made offenders particularly vulnerable when external factors threatened the status quo. We have also observed how the interaction between the borderline defensive structure and external objects is especially important in understanding why the offender kills. The predisposing defensive structure alone cannot fully explain murderous behaviour. The interaction between offender and victim/external object, and the intrapsychic exchanges between them via projective identification, also requires consideration. This was most apparent in the cases where the victims themselves were found to be violent. In discussing the dimensions earlier, I used the term 'borderline situation' to emphasize that the murderous action observed here is more than simply a consequence of the offender's own personality or defensive structure.

The assessment of dangerousness may occcur through clinical or objective methods of assessment. From a psychoanalytic perspective, observations regarding interaction between assessor and offender are an important source of information for testing hypotheses related to dangerousness (Glasser, 1996). Initial countertransference responses may also yield important clues to understanding the offender's internal world. In my view, observations here are indispensable in assessing for the presence of the intrapsychic dimensions listed above. It is important, however, to emphasize that, given the brevity of most assessment encounters, countertransference impressions need to be corroborated by other sources of information such as projective tests, collateral information, court records and so forth.

A number of earlier theoretical observations have some bearing on evaluating the likelihood of rage-type murderers re-offending, a question often asked following the crime. First, I have argued that catharsis, or the unburdening of aggressive psychic energy, does not adequately account for the complexity of object relations and the particular nature of interaction that precedes the act. Specific object selection, representational capacity and interactional patterns are not given adequate emphasis when explosive affect is conceptualized in this way. Furthermore, this has implications for the rehabilitation and prognosis of such individuals. If the rage experienced here is formulated solely as a massive catharsis, rather than being linked to a particular situation or internal object, then the prognosis will be viewed as much worse. If, on the other hand, a particular object relation is isolated in the precipitation of violence, as is being argued here, management and ideas regarding prognosis are able to be far more specific and the likelihood of re-offence is thought to be far less (Meloy, 1992).

The extent to which rage attacks are understood as being motivated by the re-enactment of past conflicts also has some bearing on re-offence. Re-enactment of conflict is often taken to be a given in understanding violence from a psychoanalytic perspective and certainly is clearly evident in a number of different forms of violence (Biven, 1997; Bollas, 1995; Hyatt-Williams and Cordess, 1996). In some of the cases previously explored there is some evidence that murder follows a particular pattern that constitutes a re-enactment. However, in my view this is often not observable, suggesting that the defensive murder is more a manifestation of a breach in usual patterns or re-enactments. I am referring here specifically to defensive patterns that serve, in phantasy, to uphold the ideal good self. In this sense, and in agreement with Ruotolo (1968), the act constitutes the emergence of a new immediate solution that differs from old forms of re-enactment. In other words, the murder represents a desperate attempt to move away from the repetition of denied conflicts that have begun to escalate. This is more typical of what Bromberg (1961) calls a new 'creative' response to what feels to be an impossible entrapping situation.

Finally, can anything be said about qualitative or quantitative differences between violence and murder? Is it simply a matter of extremes, where rage-type murder constitutes the ultimate act of violence? Such questions are important in determining whether minor acts of violence would eventually lead to murder. The assumption behind conceptualizing all forms of violence on a continuum, with murder at the extreme, implies that all individuals prone to outbursts of rage would, if pushed to their limit, ultimately kill. If this were the case, one would expect that rage-type murderers would have a history of intermittent outbursts of rage. Whilst this may be a correct assumption for some violent individuals, it is not supported in the cases of rage-type murder explored here. If only tentatively, this suggests, that qualitative differences exist between rage-murder and other acts of violence that do not end in murder. It does not follow then that individuals prone to intermittent bouts of rage would necessarily be more prone to committing murder. More importantly, findings regarding the intrapsychic dimensions of rage-type murder indicate that the act is not an inevitable endpoint solely determined by an unconscious wish or repetition. The act is dependent on a multitude of factors – internal and external – coming together at a particular time. As Hyatt-Williams (1998) points out, many individuals with similar personality characteristics may go though life without committing murder if these factors do not constellate in a way that feels unbearable or 'life threatening' to the individual.

Psychotherapeutic concerns

Rage offenders are masters at imitating external reality and heeding others' perceptions and needs in a way that makes them appear relatively unproblematic and stable. Although they often appear thoughtful and considerate, much of the time they have learned to walk through life in rather mindless and depersonalized ways. Mindlessness is essentially a means of protecting themselves from parts of the self that have either been deadened by trauma or haunted by a daunting sense of absence and 'nothingness'. Importantly, however, although rage-type offenders make use of simulation and imitation as a means of defence, this process is not perverted in the sense that it is intentionally deceptive and manipulative.

Unfortunately most of the time we only encounter such individuals after a crime has been committed. Given the overcontrolling nature of the personality they are seldom accessible to guidance or assistance. The thought of seeking help is also associated with unbearable shame.

In the cases when psychotherapy is possible, before or after the event, emphasis should be placed on facilitating a process of psychic digestion (of the bad-object system as conceptualized here) and the gradual move towards depressive experience – the depressive position – in this area of the personality. Hyatt-Williams

(1998) has written at length about the therapeutic problems encountered here. It is not my intention to explore clinical elements of the treatment process in detail here. Although issues of management and technique require considerable elucidation, I shall only outline some broad observations that relate to my understanding of the treatment process and the obstacles that require attention if progress is to be made.

Poor representational capacity

Poor representational capacity often makes psychotherapy an arduous and frequently painful task. The use of the symbolic function and a sense of perspective are often relatively absent, making communications concrete and one dimensional. Given that symbolic communications form such an important part of the therapeutic process, poor representational capacity tends to retard the therapist's ability to help. This often leads to an early impasse in the therapeutic process, leaving the therapist feeling quite helpless. Sometimes problems with mentalization and representation are taken to be a function of the individual's intellectual level or the result of some chronic incapacity in the psyche. If this is simply accepted as a given, the therapist takes to engaging merely at this level with the patient and little attempt is made to help develop this capacity.

The development of this capacity requires that the therapist be far more active in trying to get the patient to see other perspectives on his or her own communications. Interpretations proper are not useful until some degree of potential space is established. In theory, the aim here is to establish a rudimentary sense of a 'third object' being present in the room so that mental space is 'opened up' instead of 'closed down'. There are a number of technical issues that I have found useful in attempting to facilitate this process. First, poor representational capacity does not always stem from incapacity; it may also stem from psychic pain. Here the inability to think in the presence of an other is a key part of the problem. Unless the therapist is able to hold this somewhere in his or her mind in a way that leads to a sense of caring, he or she will be unable to help such offenders. This is important, although not easy, given that we are referring to offenders who have acted with extreme violence, sometimes killing others. Countertransference disclosure may also sometimes be useful when the therapeutic process has reached an impasse (Cartwright, 1997). With particular reference to the problem of poor representational capacity, disclosure serves a dual function. First, through the therapist or analyst disclosing his or her own states of mind he or she offers the patient an opportunity to see how others are able to reflect on their own mental functioning. Second, the act of disclosing also allows the therapist to assert his or her own separateness, an important forerunner to symbolic communication. Of course, countertransference disclosure is limited in its usefulness and should only be used in situations where the therapist has not lost sight of the defensive role that disclosures can sometimes play. A third technical issue that might be useful in helping develop representational capacity relates to the therapist's role as a translator, rather than an interpreter. Here, putting words to concrete feelings and thoughts essentially serves as an aid to the patient's own cognitive abilities. The introduction of basic metaphors that help consolidate the offender's thinking may also be useful here.

Working with the murder

Often rage offenders readily acknowledge the murder or act of violence and are able to verbalize some sense of loss and regret. It is very easy to be taken in by this approach and identify this as part of a process of genuine mourning. This is especially so, given that there is nothing manipulative or dishonest about the offender's convictions here. As a result the murder itself is often discussed for a couple of sessions and then left behind. Most of the time when this occurs we simply collude with the offender's convincing 'pseudo-digestive' capacities. The murder is discussed and the offender remains convinced of his or her ongoing regret and remorse.

There are often a number of clues that help identify the work of the idealized self and its pseudo-digestive capabilities. First, and most obviously, although regret is verbalized, excessive blame is placed on the victim or surrounding situations. Often, however, outright expressions of blame are rare and clues are more subtle. Second, the offender is also unable to give the therapist a clear, albeit crude, sense of *why* the offence occurred. More importantly, when one listens to accounts of the crime, there is seldom a narrative present that allows the offender to place himself at the scene and see himself as 'bad', violent, murderous and responsible for his own actions. Third, elements of the crime scene are frequently omitted or denied. Finally, the crime and victims are discussed in an idealized and unreal way.

The above are all clues that suggest that real mourning is impossible simply because they all suggest that the offender has not been able to identify, or take back, parts of himself that are damaging or have been damaged. Such a process may take a considerable amount of time, and as Hyatt-Williams indicates, in many cases mourning will always be incomplete given the extreme nature of the crime and the indigestible nature of the offender's internal world. It is important, however, that the therapist make a start in facilitating this process by not being taken in by pseudo-digestive capabilities.

Actively bringing the offender back to the murder or crime is an important start. If a patient is being treated post-offence, events related to the crime often serve a useful means of identifying different parts of the self in a memorable and identifiable way. In my view, this serves two important functions. First, it facilitates a process where the offender is truly able to recognize parts of the bad-object system, the beginnings of realizing that there is depth and a history behind the much-denied 'bad' self. Equally importantly, but often less acknowledged, offenders themselves are usually traumatized by the murder. They often experience traumatic repetitions of the murder itself either in flashbacks, or in the form of nightmares that have no symbolic value and lack associations. If these aspects are not addressed by reworking the murder scene, the traumatizing experience only serves unconsciously to reaffirm for offenders the need to split off associated parts of the self.

Transference and countertransference

Transference–countertransference interaction may display some distinctive qualities in the treatment of rage offenders. The therapist may often experience bouts of passivity and associated boredom. As well as this being a response to poor representational capacity, countertransference states of this kind can also be induced by the patient's overcontrolling defences that work to paralyse anything that exists 'outside' his or her narcissistic conception of the world. This parallels the individual's internal approach to the management of bad objects. It is also important, however, to recognize that boredom may also be part of the therapist's defensive reaction to unbearable thoughts of murder and violence. This kind of defensive reaction, if not attended to, only serves to reinforce the offender's unconscious belief that bad parts of the self need to be split off and disowned. If the therapist is to help the offender a great deal of countertransference processing is required so that he or she is able to think about the bad, murderous part of the self in a different, less defended way.

Although the therapist may be at risk for 'acting out' anger and hostility related to the crime, the level of hostility experienced here is usually not as extreme as one would first imagine. This appears related to the self-preservative or 'tragic' nature of crime. The offender's use of submissive and over-obliging strategies also tends to engender sympathy rather than anger in the therapist. Anger in the counter-transference most often needs greater attention when dealing with individuals who have intentionally inflicted suffering on others.

The other countertransference response that requires particular attention relates to is the offender's use of projective identification, and associated idealization and denial. Given the great difficulties and sensitivities the patient has with 'negative' experience, combined with the need to draw external objects into playing a part in the defensive system, the therapist may easily find him- or herself getting caught up in imitating the offender's defensive style. As alluded to earlier, the therapist may also have to contend with transference characterized by the manic takeover of the therapeutic function where the offender has adopted fixed ideas about the therapeutic process and becomes preoccupied with thoughts of how best to 'help' the therapist. There is often also a great need to search for the 'correct' responses to the therapist's comments. Although some degree of collusion is required here if the therapist is to establish a workable therapeutic relationship, the therapist has to be cautious of blindly mistaking such defensive strategies for authentic attempts at resolution. If some resolution to this transference state is achieved, the offender has to come to terms with the irony that real engagement cannot take place unless there is some degree of disengagement and independence of thought. Usually signs of blind collusion with the defensive organization occur when the therapeutic relationship is overly idealized and the therapeutic process continues unmitigated by conflict or difficulty.

Rationalizations of 'goodness'

Rationalizations that idealize achievements; behaviour and thoughts that aim to evoke an idealizing response; rigidly held righteous beliefs; over-obliging and submissive strategies; fantasies that place the symbiotic couple as separate and protected from others; and an overstated sense of benevolence are typical manifestations of the idealized self. The defensive nature of the idealized self has a number of implications for technique. Clearly, the way the therapist deals with the patient's defensive exterior depends on how one formulates the case and how one understands its functioning. The idealized self functions to ward off dangerous experience. It is believed by the patient to represent the self in its entirety and is the basis on which most achievements have been based. With this in mind, the therapist needs to exercise some caution in challenging these beliefs and ideas. That is, until the patient is able to think about himself in different ways and, in so doing, have other internal resources to rely on.

We have seen in some of the cases explored how offenders are often quick to identify signs of 'goodness' and success in the therapist as a means of establishing a symbiotic transference where projective identifications are used as a means of upholding the idealized exoskeleton. Although, at an oedipal level, this may be understood as an attempt to compare and compete in a rivalrous way, more therapeutic success is to be gained in approaching the defensive self by working with its narcissistic core.

Kohut's ideas about the mirroring and idealizing transference are useful here. Although the basis of his theory is not in keeping with the idea that narcissistic aspects of the personality are essentially defensive, as is the case with my formulation, his thoughts regarding technique provide an important means of consolidating a workable therapeutic alliance in the initial part of the treatment process. In my view, some degree of empathic mirroring needs to occur, in recognition of the offender's idealized self, before successful interpretation of defensive structures can occur. If not recognized, or prematurely challenged, interventions simply lead to increased defensiveness and further inflation of the idealized self.

Understanding the idealized self as being supported by a battery of projective identifications has a number of implications for technique. The mechanism of projective identification appears to demonstrate best how the idealized object system is held 'outside' the self, constantly making use of interaction to uphold its existence. Unless the offender is able, in a contained therapeutic environment, to 'take back' these parts of the self in a way that makes them more amenable to reality testing and depressive experience, attempts at working with the encapsulated part of the self will not succeed. Sometimes, however, this is done with great difficulty because the very ability to recognize and think about disowned objects has itself been disowned through projection. In other words, parts of the offender's preconceptive ability is disowned. Here the rigid use of projective identification in narcissistic disorders helps explain how difficult it is for such individuals to reverse the process of projection (Cartwright, 1998).

Working with the bad-object system

The encapsulated 'bad' self does not appear in a discrete form separate from other parts of the personality. However, only once the patient or offender has been able to relinquish some of his or her idealizing capabilities can he or she begin to mourn what has been lost or damaged in order to gain some ground in seeking resolution in the depressive position. If this is to be achieved the therapist has first to meet some success in containing toxic and unbearable mental states associated with shame. Some caution is needed here. As we have seen, violence is closely linked to the shameful exposure of the defensively internalized bad-object system. Having said that, in my experience I find there is generally little threat of violence in the therapeutic setting. We have seen that an ongoing escalating situation plays an important role in weakening exoskeletal defences. This, combined with the deeply encapsulated nature of the 'bad' self, makes violence unlikely in the thera-peutic setting. The danger here is related more to overexposing the offender to this part of the self in a way that does not facilitate mourning but rather encourages greater defensiveness. Often, in my view, overly structured anger-management programmes are at risk of doing this. Such programmes, especially those that are particularly brief, underestimate the encapsulated nature of the bad-object system and the need to work with the defensive organization. Because of this, the dictum that anger should be constructively expressed only leads to a kind of *manufactured* anger in such individuals which, in turn, feeds into an idealized conception that the expression of anger resolves a deeply entrenched internal situation. In short, such an approach simply bolsters narcissistic defences and achieves little by way of movement towards the depressive integration of the bad-object system.

Prevention

Observations regarding the collapse of the narcissistic exoskeleton, the exposure of the unarticulated bad-object system, intrusive identification, and the unbearable shame related to this, hopefully sheds some light on how intrapsychic mechanisms are involved in murderous action. This internal sequence of events, however, often occurs at great speed leaving very little time for any preventive action. Clearly astute assessment is an important part of setting preventive measures in place. If the therapist is successful here, prior to escalation, much work is needed to raise the potential offender's awareness of links between denied distress and the poten-tial for violence. If the therapist is in some way able to engage him here, impulsive violence stands a chance of being reduced.

Too often, however, potential signs of violence are identified retrospectively only after the crime. In my view, therapeutic intervention after the catathymic process has been set in motion is often of little help. This is mainly because the psyche is at risk of being flooded with dangerous paranoid experience and the therapist is often perceived as being a conspiring bad object. Containment is felt to be entrapping rather than soothing. This is particularly so in the non-structured environment of the therapeutic session. Further, the collapse of representational capacity, particularly in this distressed state, makes psychotherapeutic intervention difficult. For this reason therapeutic engagement at this point is often not productive and may only confuse the potential offender further.

Assuming that some indication of a potential violent situation is recognized, first-line interventions should rather concentrate on extra-therapeutic measures. Such measures would include the removal of the individual from the situation that he or she experiences as dangerously entrapping. This may, at times, require timeous interventions from other parties, such as the police or social welfare agencies. Clearly the removal of any potential weapons would also be a priority. At this point, when the offender can no longer distance him- or herself from the situation and concrete thinking takes over, the clinician or other agencies are most useful in acting as a 'third object' in attempting to extricate the individual from a spiralling pathway to violence.

Bibliography

Abraham, K. (1927) *Selected Papers in Psycho-analysis*, London: Hogarth Press.

Abrahamsen, D. (1973) *The Murdering Mind*, New York: Harper & Row.

American Psychiatric Association (APA) (1994) *Diagnostic and Statistical Manual of Mental Disorders; fourth edition, text revision*, Washington, DC: American Psychiatric Association, 2000.

Anderson, R. (1997) 'Putting the boot in: violent defences against depressive anxiety', in D. Bell (ed.) *Reason and Passion: A Celebration of the Work of Hanna Segal*, London: Duckworth.

Angermeyer, M.C. and Matschinger, H. (1996) 'The effect of violent attacks by schizophrenic persons on the attitude of the public towards the mentally ill', *Social Science and Medicine* 43: 1721–28.

Barends, A., Western, D., Byers, B., Leigh, J. and Silbert, D. (1990) 'Assessing affect-tone of relationship paradigms from TAT and interview data', *Psychological Assessment: A Journal of Consulting and Clinical Psychology*, 2: 329–32.

Bateman, A. (1996) 'Defence mechanisms: general and forensic aspects', in C. Cordess and M. Cox (eds) *Forensic Psychotherapy: Crime, Psychodynamics and the Offender Patient, Vol. I, Mainly Theory*, London: Jessica Kingsley.

Bateman, A. (1998) 'Thick- and thin-skinned organisations and the enactment in borderline and narcissistic disorders', *International Journal of Psycho-analysis*, 79: 13–26.

Bateman, A. (1999) 'Narcissism and its relation to violence and suicide', in R.J. Perelberg (ed.) *Psychoanalytic Understanding of Violence and Suicide*, London: Routledge.

Bergaret, J. (1984) 'Genealogie de la destructivité', *Revue Française de Psychanalyse*, 15: 1021–36.

Bion, W.R. (1957) 'Differentiation of the psychotic and non-psychotic personalities', *International Journal of Psycho-analysis*, 35: 266–75.

Bion, W.R. (1958) 'On arrogance', *International Journal of Psycho-analysis*, 39: 144–6.

Bion, W.R. (1959) 'Attacks on linking', *International Journal of Psycho-analysis*, 40: 308–15.

Bion, W.R. (1962a) *Elements of Psychoanalysis*, London: Heinemann.

Bion, W.R. (1962b) *Learning from Experience*, London: Heinemann.

Bion, W.R. (1963) *Elements of Psychoanalysis*, London: Heinemann.

Bion, W.R. (1970) *Attention and Interpretation*, London: Tavistock Publications.

Biven, B.M. (1977) 'A violent solution', *Psychoanalitic Study of the Child*, 32: 327–52.

Biven, B.M. (1997) 'Dehumanization as an enactment of serial killers: a sadomasochistic case study', *Journal of Analytic Social Work*, 4(2): 23–49.

Blackburn, R. (1971) 'Personality types among abnormal homicides', *British Journal of Criminology*, 37: 166–78.

Blackburn, R. (1983) 'Psychometric and personality theory in relation to dangerousness', in J.W. Hinton (ed.) *Dangerousness: Problems of Assessment and Prediction*, London: Allen & Unwin.

Blackburn, R. (1986) 'Patterns of personality deviation among violent offenders', *British Journal of Criminology*, 26: 254–69.

Blackburn, R. (1993) *The Psychology of Criminal Conduct: Theory, Research and Practice*, New York: John Wiley & Sons.

Blackman, N., Weiss, J. and Lamberti, J. (1963) 'The sudden murderer: III Clues to preventive interaction', *Archives of General Psychiatry*, 8: 289–94.

Blatt, S., Brenneis, C., Schimek, J. and Glick, M. (1976) 'Normal development and psychopathological impairment of the concept of the object on the Rorschach', *Journal of Abnormal Psychology*, 85: 364–73.

Bluglass, K. (1990) 'Bereavement and loss', in R. Bluglass and P. Bowden (eds) *Principles and Practice of Forensic Psychiatry*, London: Churchill Livingstone.

Bluglass, R. and Bowden, P. (eds) (1990) *Principles and Practice of Forensic Psychiatry*, London: Churchill Livingstone.

Bollas, C. (1995) *Cracking Up: The Work of Unconscious Experience*, London: Routledge.

Bottoms, A.E. (1982) 'Selected issues in the dangerousness debate', in J.R. Hamilton and H. Freeman (eds), *Psychiatric Assessment and Management*, London: Alden Press.

Bowden, P. (1990) 'Homicide', in R. Bluglass and P. Bowden (eds) *Principles and Practice of Forensic Psychiatry*, London: Churchill Livingstone.

Bowlby, J. (1969) *Attachment and Loss, Vol. 1, Attachment*, New York: Basic Books.

Brain, P.F. (1986) 'Alcohol and aggression – the nature of the presumed relationship', in P.F. Brain (ed.) *Alcohol and Aggression*, London: Croom Helm.

Brenman Pick, I. (1995) 'Concern: spurious or real', *International Journal of Psycho-analysis*, 76: 257–70.

Brenner, C. (1971) 'The psychoanalytic concept of aggression', *International Journal of Psycho-analysis*, 52: 137–44.

Britton, R. (1992) 'The Oedipus situation and the depressive position', in R. Anderson (ed.) *Clinical Lectures on Klein and Bion*, London: Routledge.

Britton, R. (1998) *Belief and Imagination: Explorations in Psychoanalysis*, London: Routledge.

Bromberg, W. (1951) 'A psychological study of murder', *International Journal of Psycho-analysis*, 32: 117–27.

Bromberg, W. (1961) *The Mold of Murder*, New York: Grune & Stratton.

Bucci, W. (1998) *The Application of Psychoanalytic Principles to the Treatment of Violent Adolescents*, presented at the 8th International Psychoanalytic Association Conference, London.

Buie, D.H., Meissner, W.W., Rizzuto, A.M. and Sashin, J. (1983) 'Aggression in the psychoanalytic situation', *International Review of Psycho-analysis*, 10(2): 159–70.

Campbell, D. (1999) 'The role of the father in a pre-suicide state', in R.J. Perelberg (ed.) *Psychoanalytic Understanding of Violence and Suicide*, London: Routledge.

Campbell, J.C. (1995) *Assessing Dangerousness: Violence by Sexual Offenders, Batterers, and Child Abusers*, London: Sage.

Campion, J., Cravens, J.M., Rotholc, A., Weinstein, H.C., Covan, F. and Murray, A. (1985) 'A study of 15 matricidal men', *American Journal of Psychiatry*, 142: 312–17.

Carney, F.L. (1976) 'Treatment of the aggressive patient', in D.L. Madden and J.R. Lion (eds) *Rage, Hate, Assault and Other Forms of Violence*, New York: Spectrum Publishers.

Cartwright, D. (1997) 'Some aspects of countertransference disclosure', *Psycho-Analytic Psychotherapy in South Africa*, 5: 2–23.

Cartwright, D. (1998) 'The reversal of pathological projective identifications: the problem of patient receptivity', *British Journal of Psychotherapy*, 15: 3–18.

Cartwright, D. (2000) 'Latent murderousness: an exploration of the nature and quality of object relations in rage-type murderers', unpublished doctoral dissertation, Rhodes University.

Cartwright, D. (2001) 'The role of psychopathology and personality in rage-type homicide: a review', *South African Journal of Psychology*, 31: 12–19.

Cartwright, D. (2002) 'The narcissistic exoskeleton: The defensive organization of the rage-type murderer', *Bulletin of the Menninger Clinic*, 66(1): 1–18.

Cartwright, D. and Cassidy, M. (2002) 'Working with HIV/AIDS sufferers: when good enough is not enough', *American Journal of Psychotherapy*, 56(2): 1–18.

Chasseguet-Smirgel, J. (1984) *Creativity and Perversion*, New York: W.W. Norton.

Chessick, R. (1993) *Psychology of the Self and the Treatment of Narcissism*, London: Jason Aronson.

Coid, J. (1983) 'The epidemiology of abnormal homicide and murder followed by suicide', *Psychological Medicine*, 13: 855–60.

Collins, J.J. (1989) 'Alcohol and interpersonal violence: less than meets the eye', in N.A. Weiner and M.E. Wolfgang (eds) *Pathways to Criminal Behaviour*, London: Sage.

Collins, J.J. and Bailey, S.L. (1990) 'Relationship of mood disorders to violence', *The Journal of Nervous and Mental Disease*, 178: 44–51.

Collins, J.J. and Bailey, S.L. (1989) 'Traumatic stress disorder and violent behaviour', *Journal of Traumatic Stress*, 3: 203–20.

Cox, M. (1982) 'The psychotherapist as assessor of dangerousness', in J.R. Hamilton and H. Freeman (eds) *Dangerousness: Psychiatric Assessment and Management*, London: Alden Press.

Deutsch, H. (1942) 'Some forms of emotional disturbance and their relationship with schizophrenia', in H. Deutsch (1965), *Neuroses and Character Types*, London: Hogarth Press.

Duncan, G.M., Frazier, S.H., Litin, E.M., Johnson, A.M. and Barron, A.J. (1958) 'Etiological factors in first-degree murder', *Journal of the American Medical Association*, 168: 1755–8.

Duncan, J.W. and Duncan, G.M. (1978) 'Murder in the family', in I.L. Kutash, S.B. Kutash and L.B. Schlesinger (eds) *Violence: Perspectives on Violence and Aggression*, California: Jossey-Bass.

Dura, J. (1997) 'Expressive communicative ability, symptoms of mental illness and aggressive behaviour', *Journal of Clinical Psychology*, 53: 307–18.

Emde, R.N. and Fonagy, P. (1997) 'An emerging culture or psychoanalytic research', *International Journal of Psycho-analysis*, 78: 643–51.

Exner, J.E. (1986) *The Rorschach: A Comprehensive System, Vol. 1, Basic Foundations*, New York: John Wiley & Sons.

Fairbairn, W.R.D. (1952) *Psychoanalytic Studies of the Personality*, London: Tavistock Publications.

Farrington, D.P. and Gunn, J. (eds) (1985) *Aggression and Dangerousness*, London: John Wiley & Sons.

Felthous, A.R., Bryant, S.G., Wingerter, C.B. and Barratt, E. (1991) 'The diagnosis of intermittent explosive disorder in violent men', *Bulletin of the American Academy of Psychiatry and Law*, 19: 71–9.

Fenichel, O. (1931) 'The pre-genital antecedents of the Oedipus complex', *International Journal of Psycho-analysis*, 12: 412–30.

Fenichel, O. (1945) *The Psychoanalytic Theory of Neurosis*, New York: W.W. Norton.

Fonagy, P. and Target, M. (1995) 'Understanding the violent patient: the use of the body and the role of the father', *International Journal of Psycho-analysis*, 76: 487–501.

Fonagy, P. and Target, M. (1996) 'Personality and sexual development, psychopathology and offending', in C. Cordess and M. Cox (eds) *Forensic Psychotherapy: Crime, Psychodynamics and the Offender Patient, Vol. I, Mainly Theory*, London: Jessica Kingsley.

Fonagy, P., Steele, M., Steele, H., Moran, G.S. and Higgit, A.C. (1991) 'The capacity for understanding mental states: the reflective self in parent and child and its significance for security of attachment', *Infant Mental Health Journal*, 12: 201–18.

Fonagy, P., Moran, G. and Target, M. (1993a) 'Aggression and the psychological self', *International Journal of Psycho-analysis*, 74: 471–86.

Fonagy, P., Moran, G.S., Edgcumbe, R., Kennedy, H. and Target, M. (1993b) 'The roles of mental representation and mental processes in therapeutic action', *The Psychoanalytic Study of the Child*, 48: 9–48.

Frazier, S.H. (1974) 'Murder – single and multiple', *Research Publications – Associations for Research in Nervous and Mental Disease*, 52: 304–12.

Freud, A. (1936). *The Ego and the Mechanisms of Defense*, London: Hogarth Press.

Freud, A. (1972). 'Comments on aggression', *International Journal of Psycho-analysis*, 53: 163–71.

Freud, S. (1900) 'The interpretation of dreams, part one', *Standard Edition of the Complete Psychological Works of Sigmund Freud*, 24 vols, (1953–73), (hereafter cited as *S.E.*), 4: 1–338.

Freud, S. (1905a) 'Three essays on the theory of sexuality', *S.E.*, 7: 123–243.

Freud, S. (1905b) 'Fragment of an analysis of a case of hysteria', *S.E.*, 7: 1–22.

Freud, S. (1911) 'Formulation of the two principles of mental functioning', *S.E.*, 12: 215–26.

Freud, S. (1915) 'Instincts and their vicissitudes', *S.E.*, 14: 117–37.

Freud, S. (1916) 'Some character-types met with in psycho-analytic work: III Criminals from a sense of guilt', *S.E.*, 14: 332–3.

Freud, S. (1920) 'Beyond the pleasure principle', *S.E.*, 18: 1–16.

Freud, S. (1923). 'The ego and the id', in S. Freud (1986) *The Essentials of Psycho-Analysis*, London: Penguin Books.

Freud, S. (1926) 'Inhibitions, symptoms and anxiety', *S.E.*, 20: 77–174.

Freud, S. (1933) 'New introductory lectures on psycho-analysis', *S.E.*, 22: 5–182.

Freud, S. (1937) 'Analysis terminable and interminable', *S.E.*, 23: 216–53.

Freud, S. and Breuer, J. (1895) 'Studies on hysteria', *S.E.*, 2: 1–309.

Fromm, E. (1973) *The Anatomy of Human Destructiveness*, New York: Holt, Rinehart and Winston.

Gacono, C.B. (1990) 'An empirical study of object relations and defensive operations in Antisocial Personality Disorder', *Journal of Personality Assessment*, 54: 589–600.

Gaddini, E. (1992) *A Psychoanalytic Theory of Infantile Experience*, London: Routledge.

Gallwey, P.L.G. (1985) 'The psychodynamics of borderline personality', in D.P. Farrington and J. Gunn (eds) *Aggression and Dangerousness*, London: John Wiley & Sons.

Gaylin, W. (1984) *The Rage Within: Anger in Modern Life*, New York: Simon & Schuster.

Gilligan, J. (1996) *Violence: Our Deadliest Epidemic and its Causes*, New York: Grosset/Putnam.

Glasser, M. (1978) 'The role of the superego in exhibitionism', *International Journal of Psychoanalytic Psychotherapy*, 7: 333–52.

Glasser, M. (1996) 'The assessment and management of dangerousness: the psycho-analytical contribution', *The Journal of Forensic Psychiatry*, 7(2): 271–83.

Glasser, M. (1997) 'Problems in the psychoanalysis of certain narcissistic disorders', *Psycho-Analytic Psychotherapy in South Africa*, 5: 35–49.

Glasser, M. (1998) 'On violence: a preliminary communication', *International Journal of Psycho-analysis*, 79: 887–902.

Glasser, M. (1999) 'Response to Reid Meloy: Letter to the editor', *International Journal of Psycho-analysis*, 80: 627–8.

Goldstein, J.H. (1986) *Aggression and Crimes of Violence*, London: Oxford University Press.

Goreta, M. (1990) 'The psychoanalytic approach as a contribution to the assessment of criminal responsibility', *Journal of Psychiatry and Law*, 18: 329–45.

Goreta, M. (1995) 'A contribution to the theory of psychoanalytic victimology', *Journal of Psychiatry and Law*, 23: 263–81.

Greenberg, J.R. and Mitchell, S.A. (1983) *Object Relations and Psychoanalytic Theory*, London: Harvard University Press.

Grotstein, J.S. (1981) *Splitting and Projective Identification*, London: Jason Aronson.

Guntrip, H. (1968) *Schizoid Phenomena, Object Relations and the Self*, London: Hogarth Press.

Hafner, H. and Boker, W. (1982) *Crimes of Violence by Mentally Abnormal Offenders: A Psychiatric and Epidemiological Study in the Federal German Republic*, Cambridge: Cambridge University Press.

Harris, J.E. and Pontius, A.A. (1975) 'Dismemberment murder: in search of the object', *Journal of Psychiatry and Law*, 3: 7–24.

Hartmann, H., Kris, E. and Loewenstein, R.M. (1949) 'Notes on the theory of aggression', *Psychoanalytic Study of the Child*, 3: 9–36.

Hering, C. (1997). 'Beyond understanding? Some thoughts on the meaning and function of the notion of "evil"', *British Journal of Psychotherapy*, 14(2): 209–19.

Hinshelwood, R.D. (1994) *Clinical Klein*, London: Free Association Books.

Hinshelwood, R.D. (1997) 'The elusive concept of "internal objects" (1934–43): its role and the formation of the Klein group', *International Journal of Psycho-analysis*, 78: 877–98.

Hinton, J.W. (1983) *Dangerousness: Problems of Assessment and Prediction*, London: George Allen & Unwin.

Hitchcock, J. (1996) 'Dread of the strength of the instincts', *Psychoanalytic Study of the Child*, 51: 103–16.

Hodgins, S. (1993) 'The criminality of mentally disordered persons', in S. Hodgins (ed.) *Mental Disorder and Crime*, London: Sage.

Hollin, C.R. (1989). *Psychology and Crime: An Introduction to Criminological Psychology*, London: Routledge.

Howells, K. (1982) 'Mental disorder and violent behaviour', in P. Feldman (ed.) *Developments in the Study of Criminal Behaviour, Vol. 2: Violence*, Chichester: John Wiley & Sons.

Howells, K. and Hollin, C.R. (eds) (1992) *Clinical Approaches to Violence*, New York: John Wiley & Sons.

Hyatt-Williams, A. (1996) 'Latent murderousness', *Psycho-analytic Psychotherapy in South Africa*, 4: 23–40.

Hyatt-Williams, A. (1998) *Cruelty, Violence and Murder: Understanding the Criminal Mind*, London: Jason Aronson.

Hyatt-Williams, A. and Cordess, C. (1996) 'The criminal act and acting out', in C. Cordess and M. Cox (eds), *Forensic Psychotherapy: Crime, Psychodynamics and the Offender Patient, Vol. I, Mainly Theory*, London: Jessica Kingsley.

Isaacs, S. (1948) 'The nature and function of fantasy', *International Journal of Psycho-analysis*, 29: 73–97.

Jackson, M. and Tarnopolsky, A. (1990) 'Borderline personality', in R. Bluglass and P. Bowden (eds) *Principles and Practice of Forensic Psychiatry*, New York: Churchill Livingstone.

Jacobson, E. (1954) 'The self and object world', *Psychoanalytic Study of the Child*, 9: 75–127.

Joseph, B. (1981) 'Addiction to near-death', *International Journal of Psycho-analysis*, 63: 449–56.

Joseph, B. (1997) 'Where there is no vision: from sexualization to sexuality', in D. Bell (ed.) *Reason and Passion: A Celebration of the Work of Hanna Segal*, London: Duckworth.

Jukes, A. (1993) 'Violence, helplessness, vulnerability and male sexuality', *Free Associations*, 4: 25–43.

Jukes, A. (1994) 'Working with men who are helpless, vulnerable and violent', *Free Associations*, 5: 577–603.

Kaplan, H.I. and Saddock, B.J. (1989) *Clinical Psychiatry*, London: Williams & Wilkins.

Kelly, L. (1988) *Surviving Sexual Violence*, Oxford: Polity Press.

Kernberg, O. (1966) 'Structural derivatives of object relationship', *International Journal of Psycho-analysis*, 47: 236–53.

Kernberg, O. (1980) *Internal World and External Reality: Object Relations Theory Applied*, New York: Jason Aronson.

Kernberg, O.F. (1984) *Severe Personality Disorders*, London: Yale University Press.

Kernberg, O.F. (1992) *Aggression in Personality Disorders and Perversions*, London: Yale University Press.

Khan, M.M.R. (1974) *Privacy of the Self*, London: Hogarth Press.

Kirshner, L.A. (1998) 'Challenges facing today's psychoanalytic practice', *International Journal of Psycho-analysis*, 79: 595–8.

Klein, M. (1927) 'Criminal tendencies in normal children', *British Journal of Medical Psychology*, 7: 177–92.

Klein, M. (1928) 'Early stages of the Oedipus complex', *International Journal of Psycho-analysis*, 9: 167–80.

Klein, M. (1932) *The Psycho-Analysis of Children*, London: Hogarth Press.

Klein, M. (1946) 'Notes on some schizoid mechanisms', *The Writings of Melanie Klein*, 3: 1–24.

Klein, M. (1957) 'Envy and Gratitude', *The Writings of Melanie Klein*, 3: 48–56.

Klein, M. (1958) 'On the development of mental functioning', *International Journal of Psycho-analysis*, 39: 84–90.

Kleinman, A. (1987) *Rethinking Psychiatry: From Cultural Category to Personal Experience*, New York: The Free Press.

Kohut, H. (1972) 'Thoughts on narcissism and narcissistic rage', in P. Ornstein (ed.) *The Search of the Self*, London: International University Press.

Kohut, H. (1978) *The Search for the Self*, New York: International University Press.

Konner, M.J. (1993) 'Do we need enemies?: the origins and consequences of rage', in R.A. Glick and S.P. Roose (eds) *Rage, Power, and Aggression*, London: Yale University Press.

Kutash, S.B. (1978). 'Psychoanalytic theories of aggression', in I.L. Kutash, S.B. Kutash and L.B. Schlesinger (eds) *Violence: Perspectives on Violence and Aggression*, California: Jossey-Bass.

Lacan, J. (1977) *Écrits: A Selection*, New York: W.W. Norton.

Lamberti, J., Blackman, N. and Weiss, J. (1958) 'The sudden murderer: a preliminary report', *Journal of Social Therapy*, 4: 2–10.

Lang, R.A., Holden, R., Langevin, R., Pugh, G.M. and Wu, R. (1987) 'Personality and criminality in violent offenders', *Journal of Interpersonal Violence*, 2: 179–95.

Lecours, S. and Bouchard, M. (1997) 'Dimensions of mentalisation: outlining levels of psychic transformation', *International Journal of Psycho-analysis*, 78: 855–75.

Lefer, L. (1984) 'The fine edge of violence', *Journal of the Academy of Psychoanalysis*, 12: 253–68.

Lewis, M. (1993) 'The development of anger and rage', in R.A. Glick and S.P. Roose (eds) *Rage, Power, and Aggression*, London: Yale University Press.

Limandri, B. and Sheridan, D.J. (1995) 'Prediction of interpersonal violence', in J.C. Campbell (ed.) *Assessing Dangerousness*, London: Sage.

Limentani, A. (1991) 'Neglected fathers in the aetiology and treatment of sexual deviations', *International Journal of Psycho-analysis*, 72: 573–84.

Lorenz, K. (1963) *On Aggression*, New York: Bantam Books.

McKellar, P. (1989) *Abnormal Psychology: Its Experience and Behaviour*, London: Routledge.

Meers, D. (1982) 'Object relations and beyond the pleasure principle revisited', *Psychoanalytical Inquiry*, 2(2): 233–54.

Megargee, E.I. (1966) 'Undercontrolled and overcontrolled personality types in extreme anti-social aggression', *Psychological Monographs*, 80: Whole No. 611.

Meloy, J.R. (1988) 'Violent and homicidal behaviour in primitive mental states', *Journal of American Academy of Psychoanalysis*, 16: 381–94.

Meloy, J.R. (1992) *Violent Attachments*, London: Jason Aronson.

Meloy, J.R. (1999) 'On violence: letter to the editor', *International Journal of Psycho-analysis*, 80: 626–7.

Meloy, J.R. and Gacono, C.B. (1992) 'The aggression response and the Rorschach', *Journal of Clinical Psychology*, 48: 104–14.

Meltzer, D. (1992) *The Claustrum: An Investigation of Claustraphobic Phenomena*, London: Clunie Press.

Menninger, K. (1942) *Love Against Hate*, New York: Harcourt Brace.

Menninger, K. (1966) *Man Against Himself*, New York: Harcourt, Brace and World.

Menninger, K. (1973) 'Murder (1928)', *Bulletin of the Menninger Clinic*, 37: 305–20.

Menninger, K. and Mayman, M. (1956) 'Episodic dyscontrol: the third order of stress adaption', *Bulletin of the Menninger Clinic*, 20: 153–65.

Menninger, K., Mayman, M. and Pruyser, P. (1963) *The Vital Balance: The Life Process in Mental Health and Illness*, New York: Viking Press.

Meyers, H.C. (1993) 'Two successful characterological adaptations to aggression', in R.A.

Glick and S.P. Roose (eds) *Rage, Power, and Aggression*, London: Yale University Press.

Millon, T. (1996) *Disorders of Personality: DSM-IV and Beyond*, London: John Wiley & Sons.

Milner, S.J. and Campbell, J.C. (1995) 'Prediction issues for practioners', in J.C. Campbell (ed.) *Assessing Dangerousness*, London: Sage.

Mitchell, S.A. (1993) 'Aggression and the endangered self', *Psychoanalytic Quarterly*, 62: 351–81.

Monahan, J. (1992) 'Mental disorder and violent behaviour: perceptions and evidence', *American Psychologist*, 47: 511–21.

Monahan, J. (1993) 'Mental disorder and violence: another look', in S. Hodgins (ed.), *Mental Disorder and Crime*, London: Sage.

Morrison, A.P. (1989) 'Shame, the underside of narcissism', in A.P. Morrisson (ed.) *Essential Papers on Narcissism*, New York: New York City Press.

Mullen, P.E. and Maack, L.H. (1985) 'Jealousy, pathological jealousy, and aggression', in D.P. Farrington and J. Gunn (eds) *Aggression and Dangerousness*, London: John Wiley & Sons.

Ogden, T.H. (1992) *The Primitive Edge of Experience*, London: Karnac Books.

Ornstein, P.H. and Ornstein, A. (1993) 'Assertiveness, anger, rage, and destructive aggression: a perspective from the treatment process', in R.A. Glick and S.P. Roose (eds) *Rage, Power, and Aggression*, London: Yale University Press.

O'Shaughnessy, E. (1981) 'A clinical study of a defensive organisation', *International Journal of Psycho-analysis*, 62: 359–69.

O'Shaughnessy, E. (1999) 'Relating to the superego', *International Journal of Psycho-analysis*, 80: 861–70.

Parens, H. (1993) 'Rage toward self and others in early childhood', in R.A. Glick and S.P. Roose (eds) *Rage, Power, and Aggression*, London: Yale University Press.

Parker, I., Georgaca, E., Harper, D., McClaughlin, T. and Stowell-Smith, M. (1995) *Deconstructing Psychopathology*, London: Sage Publications.

Perelberg, R.J. (1995a) 'A core phantasy of violence', *International Journal of Psycho-analysis*, 76: 1215–31.

Perelberg, R.J. (1995b) 'Violence in children and young adults: a review of the literature and some new formulations', *Bulletin of the Anna Freud Centre*, 18: 89–122.

Perelberg, R.J. (ed.) (1999a) *Psychoanalytic Understanding of Violence and Suicide*, London: Routledge.

Perelberg, R.J. (1999b) 'The interplay between identifications and identity in the analysis of a violent young man: issues of technique', *International Journal of Psycho-analysis*, 80: 31–46.

Pernanen, K. (1991) *Alcohol in Human Violence*, New York: Guilford.

Person, E.S. (1993a) 'Introduction', in R.A. Glick and S.P. Roose (eds) *Rage, Power, and Aggression*, London: Yale University Press.

Person. E.S. (1993b) 'Male sexuality and power', in R.A. Glick and S.P. Roose (eds) *Rage, Power, and Aggression*, London: Yale University Press.

Pihl, R.O. and Peterson, J.B. (1993) 'Alcohol/drug use and aggressive behaviour', in S. Hodgins (ed.) *Mental Disorder and Crime*, London: Sage.

Prins, H. (1990) 'Dangerousness: a review', in R. Bluglass and P. Bowden (eds) *Principles and Practice of Forensic Psychiatry*, London: Churchill Livingstone.

Retzinger, S.M. (1987) 'Resentment of laughter: video studies of the shame-rage spiral', in H.B. Lewis (ed.) *The Role of Shame in Symptom Formation*, New York: Erlbaum.

Revitch, E. and Schlesinger, L.B. (1978) 'Murder: evaluation, classification, and prediction', in I.L. Kutash, S.B. Kutash and L.B. Schlesinger (eds) *Violence: Perspectives on Violence and Aggression*, California: Jossey-Bass.

Revitch, E. and Schlesinger, L.B. (1981) *Psychopathology of Homicide*, Illinois: Charles C. Thomas.

Rey, H. (1988) 'Schizoid phenomena in the borderline', in E. Bott-Spillius (ed.) *Melanie Klein Today: Volume One*, London: Routledge.

Rosenbaum, M. (1990) 'The role of depression in couples involved in murder-suicide and homicide', *American Journal of Psychiatry*, 147: 1036–9.

Rosenbaum, M. and Bennet, B. (1986) 'Homicide and depression', *American Journal of Psychiatry*, 143: 367–70.

Rosenfeld, H. (1952) 'Notes on the psycho-analysis of the superego conflict in an acute schizophrenic patient', *International Journal of Psycho-analysis*, 33: 111–31.

Rosenfeld, H. (1971) 'A clinical approach to the psycho-analytic theory of the life and death instincts', *International Journal of Psycho-analysis*, 52: 169–78.

Rosenfeld, H. (1987) *Impasse and Interpretation*, London: Routledge.

Roth, M. (1990) 'Psychopathic (sociopathic) personality', in R. Bluglass and P. Bowden (eds) *Principles and Practice of Forensic Psychiatry*, London: Churchill Livingstone.

Ruotolo, A.K. (1968) 'Dynamics of sudden murder', *American Journal of Psychoanalysis*, 28: 162–76.

Salfati, C.G. (2000) 'The nature of expressiveness and instrumentality in homicide: implications for offender profiling', *Homicide Studies*, 4: 265–93

Satten, J., Menninger, K., Rosen, I. and Mayman, M. (1960) 'Murder without apparent motive: a study in personality disorganization', *American Journal of Psychiatry*, 117: 48–53.

Schachter, J. and Luborsky. L. (1998) 'Who's afraid of psychoanalytic research? Analysts' attitudes towards reading clinical versus empirical research papers', *International Journal of Psycho-analysis*, 79: 965–70.

Schafer, R. (1976) *A New Language for Psychoanalysis*, New Haven, Conn.: Yale University Press.

Schafer, R. (1997) *Tradition and Change in Psychoanalysis*, London: Karnac Books.

Schuster, R.H. (1978) 'Ethological theories of aggression', in I.L. Kutash, S.B. Kutash and L.B. Schlesinger (eds) *Violence: Perspectives on Violence and Aggression*, California: Jossey-Bass.

Segal, H. (1978) 'On symbolism', *International Journal of Psycho-analysis*, 59: 315–19.

Segal, H. (1991) *Dream, Phantasy and Art*, London: Routledge.

Segal, H. (1997) *Psychoanalysis, Literature and War*, London: Routledge.

Shengold, L. (1989) *Soul Murder: The Effects of Child Abuse and Deprivations*, New Haven, Conn.: Yale University Press.

Shengold, L. (1991) *'Father, Don't You See I'm Burning?'*, London: Yale University Press.

Shengold, L. (1993) *'The Boy Will Come to Nothing: Freud's Ego Ideal and Freud as Ego Ideal'*, London: Yale University Press.

Shengold, L. (1999) 'Foreword', in R.J. Perelberg (ed.) *Psychoanalytic Understanding of Violence and Suicide*, London: Routledge.

Shoham, S.G., Rahav G. and Addad, M. (1997) *Criminology: Theories and Research*, New York: Harrow & Heston.

Smith, B.L. (1990) 'Potential space and the Rorschach: an application of object relations theory', *Journal of Personality Assessment*, 55: 756–67.

Sohn, L. (1995) 'Unprovoked assaults – making sense of apparently random violence', *International Journal of Psycho-analysis*, 76: 565–75.

Solursh, L. P. (1989) 'Combat addiction: overview of implications in symptom maintenance and treatment planning', *Journal of Traumatic Stress*, 2: 451–60.

Spence, D. (1982) *Narrative Truth and Historical Truth*, New York: W.W. Norton.

Spillius (Bott), E. (ed.) (1988). *Melanie Klein Today: Developments in Theory and Practice. Volume 1: Mainly Theory*, London: Routledge.

Steiner, J. (1982) 'Perverse relationships between parts of the self: a clinical illustration', *International Journal of Psycho-analysis*, 63: 241–53.

Steiner, J. (1993) *Psychic Retreats*, London: Routledge.

Stern, D. (1985) *The Interpersonal World of the Infant*, New York: Basic Books.

Stoller, R.J. (1979) 'Fathers and transexual children', *Journal of the American Pyschoanalytic Association*, 27: 837–66.

Stone, A.A. (1993) 'Murder with no apparent motive', *The Journal of Psychiatry and Law*, 21: 175–90.

Stone, M.L. (1980) *The Borderline Syndromes*, London: McGraw-Hill.

Symington, N. (1996) 'The origins of rage and aggression', in C. Cordess and M. Cox (eds) *Forensic Psychotherapy: Crime, Psychodynamics and the Offender Patient, Vol. I, Mainly Theory*, London: Jessica Kingsley.

Tanay, E. (1969) 'Psychiatric study of homicide', *American Journal of Psychiatry*, 175: 1252–58.

Taylor, P.J. (1993) 'Schizophrenia and crime: distinctive patterns in association', in S. Hodgins (ed.) *Mental Disorder and Crime*, London: Sage.

Treurniet, N. (1996) 'Murderous guilt', in C. Cordess and M. Cox (eds) *Forensic Psychotherapy: Crime, Psychodynamics and the Offender Patient, Vol. I, mainly theory*, London: Jessica Kingsley.

Weiner, N.A. and Wolfgang, M.E. (1989) *Violent Crime, Violent Criminals*, London: Sage Publications.

Weiss, J., Lamberti, J. and Blackman, N. (1960) 'The Sudden Murderer: A Comparative analysis', *Archives of General Psychiatry*, 2: 669–78.

Wertham, F. (1937) 'The catathymic crisis', *Archives of Neurology and Psychiatry*, 37: 974–8.

Wertham, F. (1950) *Dark Legend*, New York: Doubleday and Company.

Wertham, F. (1962) *A Sign for Cain: An Exploration of Human Violence*, New York: Macmillan Company.

Westen, D. (1989) 'Are primitive object relations really preoedipal?', *American Journal of Orthopsychiat*ry, 59(3): 331–45.

Westen, D. (1991) 'Clinical assessment of object relations using the TAT', *Journal of Personality Assessment*, 56(1): 56–74.

Winnicott, D.W. (1965) *The Maturational Processes and the Facilitating Environment*, London: Hogarth Press.

Winnicott, D.W. (1971) *Playing and Reality*, New York: Basic Books.

Winnicott, D.W. (1986) *Home is Where we Start From*, Pelican: London.

Wolfgang, M.E. (1958) *Patterns of Criminal Homicide*, Philadelphia: University Pennsylvania Press.

Yarvis, R.M. (1972) 'The classification of criminal offenders through use of current psychoanalytic concepts', *The Psychoanalytic Review*, 59: 549–63.

Zulueta, F., De (1993) *From Pain to Violence: The Traumatic Roots of Destructiveness*, London: Whurr Publications.

Zulueta, F., De (1997) 'Demonology versus science?', *British Journal of Psychotherapy*, 14: 199–208.

Index

Milton Keynes UK
Ingram Content Group UK Ltd.
UKHW031149141024
449569UK00024B/946